HUMAN HORIZONS SERIES

LIVING A FULL LIFE

with learning disabilities

KENN JUPP

A Condor Book
Souvenir Press (E&A) Ltd

This book is dedicated to my son Adam and my daughter Mandy who, I am quite certain, would never allow anyone to prevent them from living a full life.

First published 1994 by Souvenir Press (Educational & Academic) Ltd,
43 Great Russell Street, London WC1B 3PA
and simultaneously in Canada

ISBN 0 285 63175 6

Photoset by Rowland Phototypesetting Ltd,
Bury St Edmunds, Suffolk

Printed in Great Britain by
The Guernsey Press Co. Ltd, Guernsey, Channel Islands

Acknowledgements

I would like to express my particular thanks to my wife, Sheila.

Thanks also to Jack Pearpoint, Marsha Forest, John and Angie Jones, Chris Gathercole, Judith Snow, Alan Tyne, John Hall, Joe Whittaker, Sue Thomas, Lorna, Martin and Hannah Forrest, Pat, Tom and Claire Dolan, Kevin Reeves, George Flynn, John O'Brien, Pete, Wendy and Nikki Crane, David and Althea Brandon, Martin Yates and Alan Coates. Their continued commitment, wise thoughts and encouragement over the years have been, and always will be, greatly valued.

Further thanks to Jack Pearpoint, Marsha Forest and John O'Brien for permission to include material on MAP and PATH from *The Inclusion Papers* published by Inclusion Press; and to Leslie and Mary Worrall for allowing their wedding photograph to be reproduced on the front cover of this book, and to Les Austin who took the photograph. Extracts from *Getting in on the Act: Provision for Pupils with Special Educational Needs* by the Audit Commission and Her Majesty's Inspectorate are Crown Copyright and are reproduced with the permission of the Controller of Her Majesty's Stationery Office.

This is life.
You are living it right now.
It is not a dress rehearsal.

Contents

Foreword

Living a Full Life is a great title for this excellent book by a caring friend and dedicated professional. Whilst it deals primarily with the lives of people who have learning disabilities, the logic and philosophy of inclusion on which it has been based can be applied to anybody's life. Despite the efforts made by traditional support services, people who have learning disabilities continue to be passed through a system which labels them, separates them, limits them and leads them into a life which is likely to become quite barren and lonely. No matter who we are, we should all have the chance to live meaningful lives; no one should be excluded from living his or her life to the full.

There is, in fact, only one prerequisite which anyone needs and that, quite simply, is to be able to breathe (and this includes those who do it with the assistance of a respirator). If you are capable of drawing breath, then you can also create (or be the motivation for others to create) opportunities to make the most of the time that you have, whilst you continue to live and breathe.

Life itself is a gift and it is given to all of us, whether we are able bodied or not so able bodied, capable or not so capable. No matter who we are, all our lives are enriched when we employ teamwork and live together as a group of interdependent people whom we call citizens. As citizens, we cluster effectively into places which we know as communities, where we learn to accept each other, feel a sense of belonging and support one another in our relationships. Loneliness is not an option in a true community. One might choose solitude for reflection, but no one chooses loneliness. Loneliness is the most dangerous epidemic of the twentieth century. The pain of enforced isolation can be so unbearable that some choose death, even at an early age. They do this in a number of ways—through a variety of addictions, membership of gangs or with diseases brought on by the stress of loneliness.

But there is an effective antidote to death by loneliness and the misery of having a narrow existence—building neighbourhoods which are based upon our new and yet very old ABCs:

- Acceptance
- Belonging
- Community

We also need to practise the three Rs with one another:

- Reinforcement
- Reaffirming
- Re-energising

We have to reinforce our humanity in all that we do, by such means as practising random kindness, recognising and showing appreciation to others for their kindness. We have to make the effort continually to devise senseless acts of caring in a world that is fast becoming infested with senseless acts of violence.

We must reaffirm what we know to be right. The golden rule is still a great guideline: when someone has shown kindness and caring, be sure to acknowledge it. Send them a card, write a short note or, in some other small way, show personal appreciation. Take the time and make the effort to affirm those tiny daily acts of goodness which we all experience and all too often allow to pass without remark.

We need to re-energise in order to build our communities of the future. We can do this by searching out people and places that exude energy and give us the strength to create neighbourhoods and communities where everyone is readily accepted. In these communities, the richness of diversity will allow all of us to live a fuller and more meaningful life. No matter what his or her ability, gender, cultural background or racial origin, each person is a gift, a talent, a citizen with a unique contribution to make.

The principles of inclusion are easy to understand but often hard to implement. Making it work becomes a lifelong journey.

This wonderfully readable book takes a simple, earth-shaking idea and walks us through days in our lives, so that we can see small beginning points—toe-holds to build healthier families and a new world.

Kenn Jupp has written a straightforward yet profound book. But beware: in the quiet humour and within the simple common sense of each chapter, you could find yourself changing your life. The book offers a vision and an invitation to be part of a new community. You join by reading and thinking about Kenn's view of the world. You join by your daily actions in making sure that you and your family are living a full life.

Jack Pearpoint and Marsha Forest
Directors, Inclusion Press and
The Centre for Integrated Education and Community,
Toronto, Ontario, Canada.

Preface

Most of the time, it is not their learning disabilities that are the real handicapping factor for many people, but others' perceptions of them. Without being aware of it, our love, care and concern for those close to us, who seem so vulnerable, can easily become the same all-embracing arms with which we unwittingly stifle their lives and opportunities. After all, they depend on us to empower and enable them, so that they can get the most out of their lives. The problem is that we have conditioned ourselves to see disability before we see ability. So often we latch onto the medical labels before we really get to know the people themselves, and we somehow automatically assume that we know what is best for them, without ever taking into account their own wishes and choices. We think of 'special' as being better, but this can be far from the truth.

This book is designed primarily for parents, advocates and professionals who are concerned with both children and adults who have learning disabilities. It has been written with the express purpose of getting you to consider more fully how you can best give support to the person for whom you care, whether he is a child or an adult and no matter how disabled he may appear to be. I hope this book will help you to develop some skills and understanding which will enable you to safeguard those who depend greatly upon you, so that they will not be excluded into special separate services which only prevent them from having the same opportunities as the rest of us to experience 'normality' in their lives. By 'normality' I mean simply participating fully in all the day-to-day events and routines that the majority of us already enjoy.

There are some deeply rooted underlying principles upon which this book has been based. Understanding and becoming fully conversant with them is extremely important if both you and the person for whom you care are to get the most out of living a full life. These principles are to do with the notion of INCLUSION and are built around the belief that everyone is entitled to the same choices, opportunities and status that many of us seem able to take for granted. They relate not only to children and adults who have learning disabilities, but to anyone whom we know to be regularly stigmatised, unfairly discriminated against and altogether undervalued. People who are from a different racial or cultural origin from our own, perhaps, or people of a different gender. People who have different sexual preferences from our own. People who dress differently from the way we do. People who have other religious beliefs. Ignorance, bigotry and discrimination are the basis for much disquiet and unhappiness in our world today and, make no mistake about it, these negative attitudes are continuously expressed and practised against those who are seen to have a disability. The ideology of INCLUSION will, I hope, help you to recognise and overcome these negative attitudes, particularly when they are being applied to your son or daughter or a person whom you love or for whom you are caring. By the same token, you will almost certainly find that you yourself will need to question and face up to your own stock of personal prejudices which you may have been cultivating quite unwittingly—prejudices which you may sometimes feel inwardly and perhaps even display outwardly towards a whole variety of people whom you stigmatise, discriminate against and generally undervalue.

The fundamental ideology which underpins this book therefore needs to be applied far more widely than just the field of disability, which is why Chapter One, 'Our World Needs Inclusion', has been written. It briefly examines the way our world is going today and shows why we need to practise the principles of INCLUSION for all people and not just specifically for the benefit of those who have learning disabilities. If, as a reader, you are anything like me, you will often tend to bypass the preamble of a newly acquired book like this and leap straight into the chapters that interest you most. On this occasion, assuming that you have read this far already, I ask you to resist the temptation to skip over chapters until you have first read Chapter One.

Please read on . . .

1 Our World Needs Inclusion

> 'Everything is changing. People are taking the comedians seriously and the politicians as a joke.' Will Rogers

I suppose I must have been about nine years old when I was first taken round the Natural History Museum. I remember seeing a rather fearsome display of black panthers, Bengal tigers, poisonous spiders, some pretty spiteful-looking scorpions and a whole variety of deadly venomous snakes. Thankfully, all these creatures had been immortalised by some unknown taxidermist and set safely at arm's length, behind huge plate glass windows. But as I wandered through each stately room and down the long, panelled corridors, I really was quite in awe of the fierce-looking, open-jowled animals that bared their teeth at me, as if they might pounce at any minute. These were the stuffed and mounted effigies of ferocious beasts that killed, savage man-eaters that put all else in fear of them. Finally, I came across two very regal-looking red velvet curtains which had been drawn together with a sign attached to them announcing, 'BEHIND THIS CURTAIN IS THE MOST DANGEROUS ANIMAL IN THE WORLD.' Of course, the temptation was far too much for the healthy curiosity of any red-blooded nine-year-old boy, and with some trepidation I pulled the curtains apart and cautiously peeked in, only to find myself staring into a large, full-length mirror.

It was an experience that has always stayed with me and it gave me a rather different, but clearer perspective on both myself in particular and my fellow *Homo sapiens* in general.

No matter how dangerous other animals may seem, without doubt it is we humans who are by far the most threatening species on this planet. Nevertheless, we seem to regard ourselves (with some arrogance, I always think) as being *the* most superior form of life. We speak of ourselves as being a *social* animal and yet we have developed a distinct lack of ability to get on even with each other. Nation against nation, white against black, Gentile against Jew, Protestant against Catholic, Christian against Muslim, heterosexual against homosexual, rich against poor, man against woman.

We have learned to compete rather than collaborate

For as long as I can remember, there has always been a war going on somewhere and for much of the time it has been difficult to understand why. Even as I write there are no less than forty wars being waged throughout the world. The fact is, we humans appear to prize **competition** above **collaboration**, and at every opportunity we seem to go out of our way to get *power over* each other, rather than to have *power with* each other. Unions and management struggle and compete with each other for power. Politicians spend their parliamentary lives scoring points off each other, until some major disaster, like a war, forces them into a coalition and then they begin to learn how to collaborate. Scientists keep new knowledge a secret from each other so that they can be the first to make a breakthrough.

Even in our everyday lives the lust for power and status is constantly evident. Doctors tend to exercise more *power over* than *power with* their patients. On the whole, they share very little information with you about what they are doing with your body and why. They keep confidential facts about yourself even from you and in general they seem to get more respect than they ever give. We see doctors as having status and *power over* nurses who in turn have status and *power over* receptionists who finally have status and *power over* you, the patient. Anyone who has confronted a receptionist, in a bid to get seen by the doctor without a proper appointment, will know exactly what I mean.

From bus conductors to government officials, the notion of *power over* as opposed to *power with* is predominant and has somehow become ingrained in our social infrastructure. As a result, flexibility, common sense and sound logic often go out of the window, only to be replaced by nonsensical and frustrating bureaucracy which, on the whole, is designed to keep the balance of power with those who already have it. Investing in the love of power rather than the power of love means that most of our time and resources will be taken up simply with maintaining our own position and self-interest. This is often done at the expense of those who can least afford it. If we were to collaborate more, we would surely find that pooling our skills, knowledge and resources would result in a much better future for everyone. Those of you who are my age, or older, will remember that throughout the Sixties the Soviet Union (as it was then known) and the United States, two major nations in our so-called civilised world, frantically **competed against** rather than **collaborated with** each other, so that just one of them (as opposed to both of them) could be the first nation to land on the surface of the Moon. Whilst Neil Armstrong was taking his 'one giant leap for mankind', literally millions of people in the Third World were in desperate need of food and shelter. What is worse is that today things are no different. Whilst half of our world is dying of starvation, the other half seems to be on the 'F' Plan Diet.

We baffle ourselves with bureaucracy

The madness that we introduce into our lives goes on. We continue to invest more in bureaucracy than we do in sound common sense. In Europe, farmers and agriculturalists have made considerable progress in developing advanced machinery and techniques in the growth and harvesting of crops, but unbelievably, at the same time they are being paid significant subsidies by the EC *not* to grow things. This same tragic logic was illustrated most graphically in 1992, when a team of Russian cosmonauts was left to orbit in outer space for an extra three months, simply because their government couldn't afford to bring them back to Earth until the beginning of their next financial year.

It would all be very funny if the results of our senselessness were not so devastating for countless others in need, with whom we share this planet. Once we start to look beyond our own front gates, it becomes painfully evident that futile actions like these are being perpetrated on a very large scale, not just at government level but by all of us, towards each other, in our everyday lives. Secretaries, telephonists, caretakers—anyone who wears a peaked cap for that matter—are just a few who, to our eternal frustration, seem to be more comfortable telling us why we can't do things rather than helping us to achieve them. That abrupt car park attendant is quick to tell us, 'You can't park there!' but slow to help us discover exactly where we can park. Even in social situations we often find ourselves practising some form of one-upmanship and discovering new ways of 'getting one over' our friends and neighbours—but why? Where have we learned this from and where is it getting us?

We need a better philosophy for our improved technology

When you start to take a long, hard look at the world, you soon find yourself in real trouble trying to figure out the logic of it all. How did we get ourselves into such a mess? How did our reasoning become so mixed up? It certainly isn't through lack of wit or ingenuity, since we have made some great strides in many other areas of achievement. In our technology, for instance, we have progressed at a tremendously rapid rate. We can now transplant vital organs, move at twice the speed of sound, communicate instantly across the world by telephone, computer networks and fax machines. We have known for years how to split the atom and we can engage in genetic engineering as if we were playing with Lego bricks.

Without question we have developed any number of clever ways of doing things, but (and here's the rub) we have neglected to formulate sound philosophies and ideologies with which we can begin to understand ourselves and our own true needs as people. As a result, we create new technologies without knowing how to apply them properly or what the implications may be. Generally speaking, we have succeeded in creating more problems than we can actually solve. Of this, Albert Einstein (who, incidentally, was unable to attend university until he was 29 years old because we told him that he didn't have the proper entry qualifications) said, 'The world which we have made, as a result of the level of thinking we have done this far, creates problems we cannot solve at the same level at which we created them.'

Today we find that, in all major aspects of our daily lives, our world seems to be at some crisis point or other. Those people who regard themselves as experts in their various fields now appear to be quite incapable of doing much about the difficulties that exist. Take ecologists, for instance. They are struggling with the problem of pollution, which by all accounts is getting more and more out of hand as time goes on. By the same token, policemen are unable to detect crime at the rate at which it is now being committed. This, we are told, is at epidemic proportions and still rising. Our prisons are overcrowded and our penal system is straining under the weight of responsibility in trying to keep ever-increasing numbers of offenders from continuing to offend. Added to this, doctors remain at a loss to know how to cure the common cold, let alone deal with the threat of AIDS. Economists keep telling us that an end to our financial recession is just around the corner, yet a record number of businesses persist in sliding into bankruptcy, and unemployment seems to be the only real growth industry that we can manage to sustain. Our pharmaceutical and medical expertise has brought about wide use and availability of narcotics, which has spawned a scale of drug abuse that is proving impossible to control. As far as housing is concerned, more people than ever live in what our estate agents would no doubt describe as 'compact bijou residences located in the fashionable part of town, overlooking the Thames'. We of course know them as cardboard boxes.

So for all our technology, in real terms our quality of life is relatively poor these days. Even with our houses securely locked and barred, few of us go away for any length of time without experiencing some unease about what we might find when we get back. I, for one, am beginning to understand that it doesn't have to be this way. We can all live better and fuller lives. We can begin to harness the advantages of our technological advancements if we develop a sound philosophy to implement as a basis for good living. We cannot change the whole world tomorrow, of course, but we can each change a little bit of it every day.

We are each responsible for how things are

It would be most unwise of us to bury ourselves in smug complacency, thinking that all these downward trends will one day magically disappear without any effort on our part. Whether we like it or not, the sort of world in which we now live is the direct result of our own accumulated efforts. Each of us has made a personal contribution to the lifestyle that we are experiencing today. The consequences of our combined individual actions, values and beliefs shape our planet, our nations, our local communities and, ultimately, our relationships with one another. Surely the time is long overdue for us to make some fundamental changes to the way we think and the way we live.

Making changes is not nearly so difficult as some people would have us believe. The fact is, nothing stays the same anyway. In this world, change is guaranteed; it's the one thing that you can really rely upon. No matter what you do, you can't stop it. What is important is how we make these changes. But before we can expect to change others, we have to begin by changing ourselves; we have to have a shared philosophy, principles that would enable us to live with one another in a way that benefits us all. The ideology of INCLUSION is now fast becoming a rationale which is being promoted around the world. It encompasses all that is necessary for us to turn our moral, financial and physical descent into an upward trend. So what are these principles of INCLUSION?

A QUICK AND EASY ALPHABETICAL REFERENCE TO THE PRINCIPLES OF INCLUSION

'There is in this world today, a vibrant new culture. It is young and rough, but with proper nurturance, its life and growth promise to be dramatic. It is the culture of INCLUSION.'

Judith Snow

A is for ACCEPTANCE

We need to start accepting each other for who we are and what we are, otherwise we will continue to ruin lives from the effects of our own prejudices, discrimination and bigotry.

B is for BELONGING

Everyone belongs, irrespective of their looks, their gender, their physical and intellectual ability, their race, their religion or their sexuality. No one should be left out of our community.

C is for COMMUNITY

Together we are better. In our families, in our circles of friends, locally, regionally, nationally and internationally, communities of people that collaborate and support each other, in both work and play, build better futures.

D is for DIVERSITY
Categorising and labelling people in order to place them apart from everyone else means that we all miss out on the gifts that we might otherwise share. The diversity of cultures, ideas, abilities and skills, when shared, enriches life for everyone.

E is for EMPOWERMENT
Accumulating and maintaining power for ourselves means that we become defensive and anxious to keep it. But sharing our knowledge, skills and resources empowers us all.

F is for FEELINGS
Feelings are better when they are expressed. Without them, we are dead.

G is for GIFTS
Everyone has gifts to share, but they are not always readily recognised and appreciated. Those, for example, who are extremely physically weak have the ability to bring out the caring side of those who are physically strong.

H is for HUMOUR
Without humour, when would we ever laugh?

I is for INVITATIONS
Often strangers may seem a little distant and reluctant to get involved. Sometimes, all that is needed is your invitation in order to find out how delighted they are to respond.

J is for JUSTICE
Justice has to be regarded as a basic right for everyone, no matter who we are, so that we all have an entitlement to the same choices, opportunities and status that most of us already seem able to simply take for granted.

K is for KINDNESS
It is far better to receive kindness than cruelty, so why give anything else?

L is for LOVE
Without love we only exist. Each of us needs to be in touch with our own feelings, and the best feeling by far is one of love.

M is for MIRROR
Each one of us needs to use some form of mirror from time to time, so that we can see ourselves as other people see us and reflect upon the way we are.

N is for NEEDS
One of our greatest needs is to be able to recognise our own and other people's true needs.

O is for OPPORTUNITY
We need continually to create as many opportunities as we can, for ourselves and others, and to be sure that we take full advantage of them.

P is for PEOPLE
People must always be recognised and treated as people first, whatever package they may come wrapped up in.

Q is for QUESTIONS
If we are to grow in our understanding, then it is essential for us continually to question ourselves and others about what we are doing and why.

R is for RESPECT
Respect for ourselves, in order that we in turn can be respected by others. And respect for others, so that they in turn can have respect for themselves.

S is for SUPPORT
No matter how strong we may seem, there will always be times when we need someone to lean on.

T is for TOLERANCE
Tolerance of others, whom at first we may not always completely understand.

U is for UNDERSTANDING
Without which prejudice, discrimination and bigotry rule supreme.

V is for VALUES
Values are born of the beliefs we hold, the vision we share and the dreams we dream. Our values reflect who we are and help us to live a fuller life.

W is for WELCOME
A welcome can easily be extended to everyone, simply by the light in our eye, the smile on our face and the unlimited width of our open arms.

X is for XENIAL
This is a word which means hospitable. In offering our hospitality we open doors that might otherwise remain closed. This way we can begin to discover the importance of the equation which states that the love which we take must be equal to the love that we make.

Y is for YOU
From where change begins.

Z is for ZEAL
It is zeal that fuels our actions and gives us the energy to go on.

The inclusion of people who have additional needs

Engaging these simple concepts means that, as a society, we can begin to meet our own needs at the same time as meeting other people's. If we are to curb our rising crime rate, overcome pollution and learn how to live with each other in peace and harmony, then beginning to address these principles is a good place to start. They make a firm foundation on which to build our human services, as they will ensure that in the future people will no longer become marginalised, undervalued or excluded.

On the face of it, our various education authorities, and our health and social services, seem to be very caring and responsible when it comes to providing for those people in our society who are particularly vulnerable. People who find it difficult to manage routine tasks without a considerable amount of help. People who have physical disabilities, mobility constraints, sight or hearing impairments, or perhaps a combination of these. People who become ill, physically and mentally. People who lack stability in their own emotional wellbeing. People who have learning difficulties and need the support of others to enable them to have equal opportunity. Without doubt, as a society we certainly do attempt to care for these people and already invest considerable effort, time and resources in a whole range of services which are specifically designed to improve their quality of life.

Unfortunately, even with the best of intentions, our efforts, until now, have fallen somewhat short of the mark. We have unwittingly relegated some people to a second-class human league by continually concentrating on 'doing things to them' rather than 'enabling and empowering them' to live the lifestyle of *their* choice. Somehow, we have become rather adept at mystifying the additional needs of certain children and adults. These, we say, are people who need specialist help, specialist staff, special places; but these 'special' places simply turn out to be places which are in fact separate, which segregate them from everyone else. Those people whom we call 'special' are the ones we earmark for a life apart.

We can so easily forget that those of us who have additional needs also have all the same basic human needs as anyone else. Whoever we are, we need to give and receive love, develop friendships, support each other, and have the same learning opportunities and fundamental experiences. If any of us were placed in an environment where few others talked, where we were guarded and given little choice or opportunity (all done for 'our own protection'), where we were separated from our family and friends and made to appear somehow different from everyone else, then it would be wholly unsurprising if, as a result, our performance, development and wellbeing became significantly impaired. Without realising it, special schools, group homes and institutions restrict rather than enhance the lives of those who have additional needs. Above all, irrespective of the degree of his or her disability, your son or daughter needs to be part of the everyday life of the local community. What is more, the local community needs them to be a part of it too. For these people, the notion of INCLUSION, therefore, is largely about shifting paradigms, as shown in Figure 1.

Changing how we perceive and present some people

This book is therefore largely about why and how you should resist what segregated services and 'special' places have to offer, as these inevitably lead to restrictions, isolation, fewer opportunities and, in general, an unfulfilled life. We should find it easy to identify with those who have additional needs since all of us are likely to experience some similar needs in our own lives from time to time, although of course there is a vast difference between our temporary incapacities and other people's permanent disabilities. Nevertheless, we know what it is like to experience depression or feel a little paranoid sometimes, or to find ourselves in a situation where

WE NEED TO MOVE AWAY FROM.....	AND MOVE TOWARDS.....
Separating people into special places.	Including people into everyday routines, situations and events, within their local neighbourhood.
Empowering professionals and paid staff.	Empowering users of services and their families.
Categorising people in order to fit them into an existing service.	Finding out what is really disabling the person and design a system of support which will enable them.
Artificially consigning people to special groups.	Expanding people's opportunities to develop wider social contacts and community networks.
Responding bureaucratically to control from the top.	Changing those structures which limit us.
Focusing on what is.	Focusing on what could be.
Building special units, special clubs, special schools and special projects.	Building relationships and a sense of community.
THIS WAY LEADS TO......	**THIS WAY LEADS TO......**
PREJUDICE AND CLIENTHOOD	**BELONGING AND CITIZENSHIP**

Figure 1. *Shifting paradigms.*

we have to confront a minor phobia, without being considered mentally ill. Accidents resulting in fractured bones may temporarily impose upon us some awareness of other people's mobility difficulties. Being unable to converse in a foreign country is an experience that will highlight, to some extent, the frustration of being unable to communicate properly or make our thoughts and needs known. At any given time, we can find ourselves in a situation where *we* become the ones who have additional needs.

The notion of ability and disability is in fact quite relative and exists largely in the eye of the beholder. Depending on your own standpoint, what one person would regard as quite able, another would see as quite unable. The same applies to old and young, rich and poor, big and small—they are all concepts which are relative to where we see ourselves on the continuum.

Unfortunately, the services we have developed to date have on the whole portrayed people who have additional needs as a 'species' quite different from the rest of us. Some professionals see them as a group who must be labelled and collected together under the same roof so that they can be protected from the outside world and 'treated for the condition they are in' at the same time. Similarly, tin-shakers and high-profile fund-raisers quite unwittingly see to it that those who are the subject of their good intentions become the recipients of charity rather than being afforded their rights. Telethons and sponsored events certainly raise the necessary cash, but at whose expense and whose cost? They do little for the dignity of those who are the receivers, but a good deal for the image of those who are seen to give. The media too takes its toll on those who have additional needs, either presenting them as dangerous and unpredictable or as pitiful but brave people.

Those who have additional needs, then, are likely to go through life isolated from the rest of us, facing other people's prejudices and discrimination. They will be continually confronted with attitudes of condescension and sometimes fear. They will have all this to contend with, over and above the effects of their disability, unless we begin to recognise this and change things now by adopting the principles of INCLUSION. This ideology emphasises the need to be aware that all people should be valued. If life is precious, then it must be regarded as precious for us all. If opportunity is important, then it must be made available equally to everyone, irrespective of their physical or intellectual ability, their appearance, their age, their gender, their racial origins, their culture or their sexuality.

2 New Life, New Hope

> 'When I was born, they thought that I was gonna die. But I fooled them all, even my parents.' Lori Bresina

Each time a baby is born, new hope comes into the world. Perhaps this child will be another Martin Luther King or another Albert Einstein. But long before they are even born, our children's quality of life is uppermost in our minds. As parents, we hold a deeply rooted conviction that, no matter what, we will always endeavour to do our utmost to ensure that our children have every opportunity to succeed in the life ahead of them. But of course, success is measured in as many different ways as there are people in the world. For some it is the accumulation of wealth and possessions; for others it may be the attainment of academic excellence or simply maintaining a secure job and a happy family life. One person may regard fame and recognition by the community at large as the desired goal, while another may strive merely to achieve peace of mind, satisfaction and fulfilment.

Whatever our criteria, the likelihood is that our children will measure success quite differently. Indeed, even our own set of values tends to change with age and experience. Whoever they are, whether they are disabled or not, our children have to become their own people, make choices according to their own tastes and be as self-determining as they can. Of course, no matter how old they get, they will always remain our children and we shall continue to feel proud of them and anxious for them, just as we did when they were young. Even so, they will never thank us for treating them as children once they are adults.

If you are a parent of someone who has a learning disability, you will undoubtedly feel a greater responsibility towards your child, as he or she can be particularly vulnerable. However, in real terms, *all* children are vulnerable and *all* children are entitled to our total care and concern. This is what makes parenting so difficult, for we not only have to recognise our duty to be protective, but must also try not to be *over*protective. Getting the balance right and keeping it right is by no means easy. Judging appropriately when to hold on and when to let go, when to speak up and when to shut up, becomes the basis for your child's growth and development, whether or not he or she has a learning disability.

Good parenting means being able to calculate the risk, for life is a succession of risks which have to be taken: at the core of every risk there is always an opportunity, and at the core of every opportunity there is always a risk. The outcome of each situation presents our children with experience and learning and determines how they shape themselves in life. We cannot live life for them, nor should we want to try. No matter how disabled they may be, throughout their lives your children will not only need to be loved, but also to be valued, empowered, given choice, have equal opportunity and, above all, be included. Sometimes it all seems such a huge task, with so much to consider and so many decisions to make, but the best advice anyone can give about good parenting can be summed up in just one word—'*relax*'.

Don't let your actions and attitudes (or anyone else's, for that matter) disable your child's life. Irrespective of his level of ability, he is first and foremost a child, with the same fundamental needs that other children have. It is all too easy to forget this once a label has been attached.

Latching on to a label

The problem with labels is that we learn, quite erroneously, to blame everything onto them. The fact that someone sits rocking rhythmically all day, or even banging his head, is more likely to do with the fact that he is bored than with his learning disability. Screaming fits do not occur simply because a learning difficulty exists but because of pain like toothache, or fear, or frustration from being unable to communicate an idea or feeling, or sometimes simply from sheer naughtiness. It is amazing how quickly and effectively young children seem to learn all the 'wrong' things.

Labels, too, may be a negative influence on our own attitudes if we allow them to be. Once we begin to see that our child is not doing the things that other children of his or her age are doing quite well, the anxiety inside begins to take hold. Finally the fears are confirmed when we are given a label for our child—'Down's syndrome', 'cerebral palsy', 'Retts syndrome', or whatever. It is strange, but at times like this parents often have a feeling of relief and, at the same time, a feeling of even greater anxiety. Relief that they no longer have to go on wondering, and greater concern because they still don't know what it will mean in precise and practical terms. Many parents seek desperately for a label. Even though it may make very little difference to the circumstances, they will at least feel less pent up by knowing exactly what they are up against.

Once the label is unveiled (although often it never is) there is a real danger that it will prejudice parents' expectations, which in turn can undermine their child's learning, opportunities, experiences and chance to live a full life. The spiral shown in Figure 2 is going in a downward direction. It starts by recognising that a child is delayed in certain areas of his or her development. This leads parents to form low expectations of their child's abilities generally, which in turn teaches the child that he is incapable. Above all, he learns that he cannot do things. This is reinforced when parents do things for him, believing their child to be quite unable to learn for himself. As a result, their child gets little or no opportunity to learn for himself and little or no motivation either. Being deprived of both opportunity and motivation, their child's experiences become greatly diminished, and for the most part the experiences he does have are quite negative ones (e.g. 'Don't do that . . . I'll do it for you'). The result of all this is the creation of greater developmental delay day by day, as their child grows older but is continually prevented from learning.

On the other hand, the spiral can be reversed and be made to go in an upward direction (see Figure 3). This spiral would start by parents breaking tasks into a sequence of easy stages so that their child can be encouraged to tackle each simple stage and be applauded for each small success. This way the child will have ever-increasing experiences and greater learning success in an open-ended spiral of endless opportunity.

Finding out and coping

How you find out that your baby has additional needs varies from place to place and person to person. In some instances, parents have said that they were never actually told at all, but simply left to become aware of it by themselves. If you give birth in a hospital, however, and your baby has a fairly easily recognisable condition like Down's syndrome, then the chances are that you will be told before leaving. Nevertheless, it could be at least a day or two before the doctor or midwife divulges the information to you.

Part of the problem for doctors in delivering the news is that they have little or no training in how to go about it. Consequently, mothers are often told without their partners present and find themselves in the unenviable position of having to break the news to their nearest and dearest on their next visit. Privacy too is often lacking. It is difficult to find a quiet, unoccupied room in a hospital, and curtains pulled round your bed in the maternity ward are usually not enough to give you all the privacy you need, although they often have to serve the purpose. Some parents have been falsely reassured and their anxious questions—'Where's my baby? Why has everyone else got theirs?'—are sometimes answered with a white lie from a well-meaning ward sister,

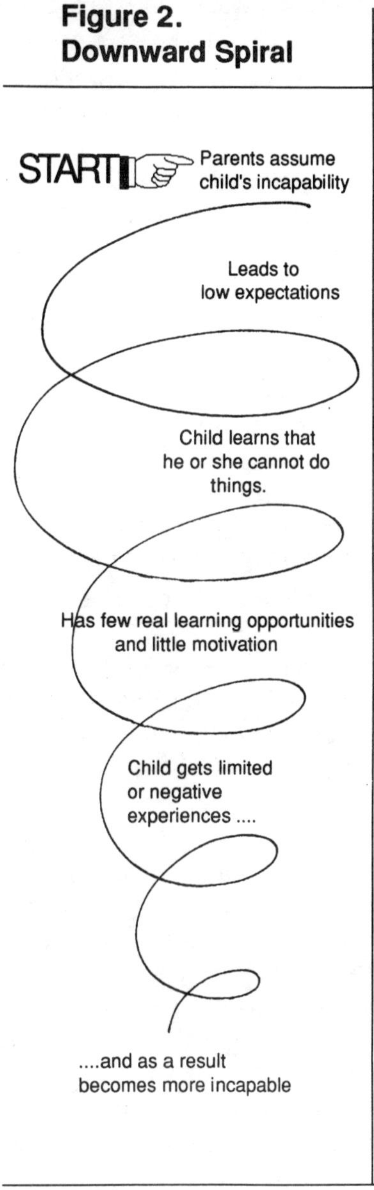

Figure 2.
Downward Spiral

Figure 2. *Downward Spiral.*

Figure 3.
Upward Spiral

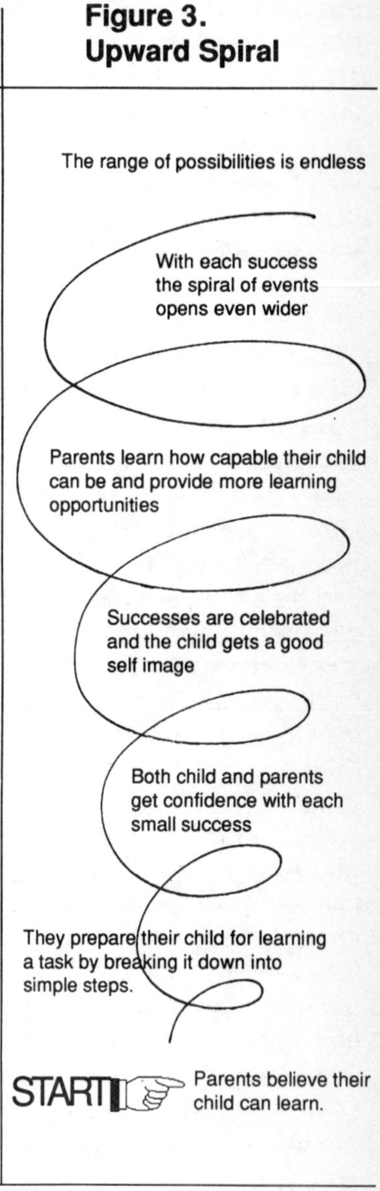

Figure 3. *Upward Spiral.*

who seeks to put the mother's mind at rest in a bid to play for time until the doctor becomes available. Many hospitals make it a rule that only the doctor is allowed to break the news. So it can be hours or even days before he or she arrives, and in the meantime the mother is told that there is nothing for her to worry about and that all is well.

It is little wonder, then, that some parents learn to mistrust doctors and nurses from day one. Of course, members of the medical profession themselves find it emotionally difficult to cope with what they perceive as irredeemable situations. Their training, after all, is geared to curing people, making them better, repairing damage. Confronting such a diagnosis, in which they know they can have only a limited effect, is therefore likely to leave them feeling powerless, ineffectual and with a certain sense of failure. At the same time parents are left feeling numb with shock. Throughout the pregnancy they have cultivated an image of a perfect child, and now they are faced with a reality vastly different from what they have been expecting.

In a recent survey parents whose babies had been born with some anomaly were asked what, in retrospect, they felt should be taken into account when disclosing an unexpected diagnosis to other parents in the future. The following are some of the replies:

1 Parents want to be informed immediately, or certainly within 24 hours if possible.
2 If it is not possible to diagnose accurately straight away, parents want to know of the doctor's suspicions rather than be fobbed off with false reassurances.
3 If doctors are in the process of carrying out tests, then parents want to know about it: what the tests are for, what is involved and how long they will take.
4 Parents want medical staff to be open, frank and honest with them.
5 Mother and father want to be told together, so that they can get support from one another.

6 Parents want privacy and some time together on their own, during and after receiving the news.
7 Parents want their baby present during and after the time of telling, so that they can see that their child has positive and attractive features, rather than being left to imagine the worst.
8 Parents would like someone else to be present as well as the doctor, so that when he or she leaves they have a knowledgeable person who can spend some time with them, going over the information and answering any questions they may have.
9 Parents want to be left with some written information about their child's condition, and addresses where they can get additional information and help.
10 Parents want doctors to use simple language and not baffle them with science.

Whilst every individual is different, there does seem to be an overall pattern to the way parents respond after they have been told. As has already been said, parents expect to have a perfect child, but some differences can be accommodated without much trouble. For instance, if a boy arrives instead of the wished-for girl, the disappointment is soon overcome. But where the discrepancy is too great, then the trauma becomes longer term. In situations like this couples have to reconstruct their whole lives as well as their baby, based upon entirely new information. Figure 4 shows how most people react after disclosure that their baby has been born with a disability.

SHOCK

Initially, there is the shock. Most parents describe a feeling of numbness when they are first confronted with the news. They experience feelings of loss—loss of the perfect baby that they had expected and loss of their hopes and dreams. It is a time of extreme pressure, when they are required to absorb and accept the reality of the situation and begin car-

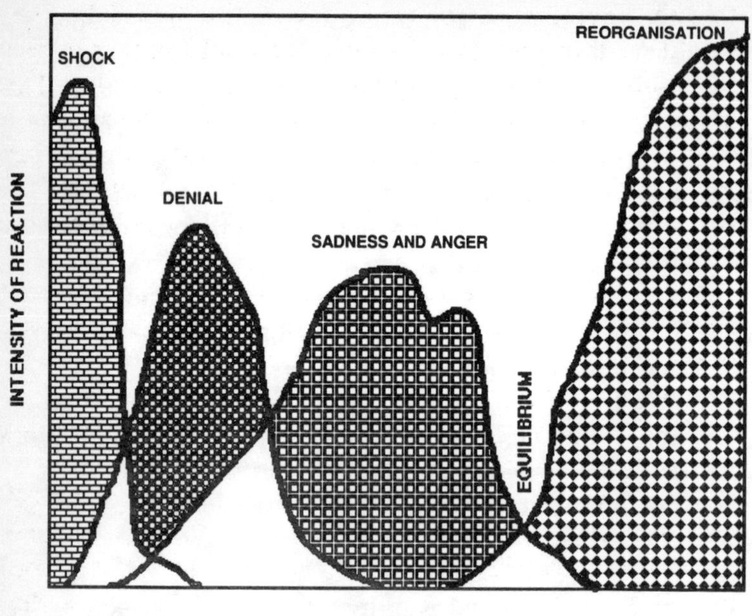

Figure 4. *Parents' emotional reactions.*

ing for their child who is to be a part of their family for the rest of their lives. At this time it is quite natural for parents to have one of two strong feelings. They may have a sense of great protection for their baby or they may feel rejection and want to 'switch off' their emotions. It is certainly not unusual for fathers in particular to feel this way.

Communication is very necessary. Make sure that you talk to your partner or the person who is close to you and share your feelings with each other. Marriages come under much more stress when couples feel unable to communicate their innermost feelings. On the other hand, relationships are made closer and strengthened when people talk frankly and honestly. Janet was born with a respiratory disorder, and had to be taken into hospital for frequent emergency treatment throughout the first two years of her life. She had a number of major disabilities and on many occasions her parents were told that her chances of survival were fifty-fifty. Then she would recover, only to go through the whole pattern of hospital admission and recovery again some weeks later. This naturally took its toll on the parents who never knew whether the next time would be Janet's last. Then, when Janet was once again taken as an emergency patient into the children's ward, with an unsure outcome, her mother came to see me.

'Don't tell my husband,' she said, 'but I hope Janet doesn't come out of it this time. I don't think I can take much more of this, and anyway, what sort of future is there for Janet?'

A while later, Janet's father visited me.

'Don't say anything to my wife,' he said, 'but I really think it's better all round if Janet doesn't make it this time.'

A week later Janet returned home healthy and both parents felt guilty about wishing their child dead. After some persuasion,they began to tell each other what they had told me. They shared their feelings, particularly the ones that they were ashamed of, and found that they became a greater source of strength to each other and grew much closer.

We know that at least 20 per cent of parents consider at some time the taking of their disabled baby's life. The figure is probably much higher. This sort of personal anxiety has to be shared with those close to them, in order to find ways of overcoming the sadness and replacing it with hope.

DENIAL

Following shock there is likely to be a period of denial when there is disbelief and questioning. Very often parents will 'shop around', looking for second opinions or alternative answers. They cannot believe that this has really happened and sometimes go to great lengths to try and prove that it hasn't. This may also be a time when some in-laws will be heard to say things like, 'Well it couldn't have come from our side of the family.'

SADNESS AND ANGER

Next, and interweaving with the other feelings of shock and denial, there is sadness and anger. This is a time of emotional confusion. Couples may feel anger at the loss of their perfect child, and this can show in aggressiveness towards helpers and professionals whom they come across, particularly the newsbreaker. It may be that the 'shopping around' period did not yield any positive results but in fact only confirmed the original diagnosis. Parents start to question themselves very deeply and become mixed up in their thoughts. Often, for one reason or another, they blame themselves. They may lack confidence in their own ability to bring up their child. Sometimes the mother has a sense of guilt because she feels she may have mismanaged her own pregnancy in some way, or sees it as some sort of punishment for things she has done in the past. These feelings are not unusual and it is important that couples share them with each other or with family or friends. Everyone needs someone to lean on from time to time and no one can cope entirely alone.

EQUILIBRIUM

Eventually there is equilibrium, when the intensity of feeling becomes less. It feels a little like the calm after the storm. Parents have very little emotional resilience and are somewhat fragile. Any additional stress, such as a complication with their baby's condition, can take them back into the feelings of shock that they experienced initially. Equilibrium is a time when parents are in fact replenishing their stock of emotional reserves, which enables them to come finally to a stage of reorganisation.

REORGANISATION

Before this stage is reached months or even years may have passed, depending upon each individual situation. Parents develop some confidence in their own abilities to care for their child and improve their self-esteem. They are now not only in a position to meet their son's or daughter's needs, but have the experience and expertise to be a source of help to others.

As Figure 4 shows, people's feelings throughout each of these stages overlap each other, and the time taken to move from one into the next may be hours, days, weeks, months or years, depending upon the individual and his or her circumstances. It is important to realise that moving through these stages is not the end of the story. Throughout your life, you as parents will be presented with new and different situations, each of which is likely to take you through these stages of feeling again—for instance, having your child statemented as having special educational needs, helping him or her through adolescence, leaving school, considering what is going to happen to him when you are no longer here. However, each obstacle that you overcome will prepare you better for the next. You will gain more experience, have greater knowledge and make more contacts and friends to help you as you go along.

Facing the dilemmas

Once you know your youngster has learning disabilities, the chances are that the difficulties you have to confront will come not so much from your son's or daughter's additional needs as from the services that are provided to meet them. As a rule of thumb, it generally pays not to get too involved with any service that has the word 'special' in its title. So often 'special' is a euphemism for 'segregated'. Special schools, special units, special classes and so on, no matter how well equipped and attractive they are, will all serve to keep your child away from ordinary everyday life experiences and from other local people. As matters stand now, parents of children who have additional needs are faced at some stage in their lives with a tremendous dilemma: they may well have to choose between meeting their child's needs themselves at home, or enrolling him or her into alternative provision away from home. It is an impossible decision that no one should have to make, a very personal and individual decision that is difficult, if not impossible, to avoid.

On the one hand, parents may feel that others who are professionally skilled can make better provision than they can themselves, and that their son or daughter would therefore have his or her needs better met if he were allowed to live apart from the family in residential accommodation. Statistics do show that a higher percentage of marriages end in divorce where there is a child in the family who has additional needs. There may be other considerations too, such as brothers and sisters. How will they get their fair share of love and attention with someone around who demands a great deal of time and effort from the family? Will their school work suffer if they cannot get a regular good night's sleep because their brother or sister has very irregular night habits? The considerations are manifold, but even so, having come to the conclusion that their child should live away, after agonising over it for months or even years, parents' stomachs still churn over in bed at night thinking of their child lying somewhere else and wondering if they have made the right decision; wrestling with their inner feelings, not knowing whether they have given their child the best opportunity or abandoned him when he needed them most.

On the other hand, some will take the view that their child must remain with them no matter what. This decision can place an incredible strain upon all members of the family. Everyone will need to make sacrifices, sometimes quite considerable ones, and as their child gets bigger and heavier, the parents get older and less able to cope. Some extremely elderly parents may still be living with and caring for their son or daughter who herself has now become a senior citizen. Most children outlive their parents and those who have learning difficulties are no different, so when parents finally die those who are left behind are taken into the very place that their parents have spent a lifetime trying to keep them away from. They lose their parents, their home and their familiar surroundings, all at the same time.

So it seems impossible to make the right decision, whatever one chooses to do. It must seem like playing Russian roulette with a fully loaded revolver. Parents cannot win, because on the one hand nobody provides families with what they really need—individual personalised extra help at home or wherever it is needed—while the guilt and uncertainty of sending a child away is often too great to overcome. On the other hand, most residential establishments are more like institutions than homes, no matter how well appointed they may be. The principles of INCLUSION can be used to overcome this two-way emotional stretch and assist parents and other interested people to plan a sound strategy that will take practical account of everyone's needs, so that children with learning disabilities and their families can have the proper support they need to enable them to live a full life.

Which road to take?

Almost as soon as your child is born you will have to make a choice about the direction in which you want to go. Will you choose the road to INCLUSION or the road to EXCLUSION? If you simply do nothing and let events take their course, before you know it you are likely to find that doctors, nurses, social workers, teachers and the like will have taken over the helm. They will make arrangements in what they will tell you are the best interests of your child. If you let them, they will also make most of the key decisions on your behalf, decisions which may well affect your lives for some time to come. Before you can say 'segregation' you may find that you have begun to travel the path of EXCLUSION, and the farther you go down this road, the harder it will become for you to turn and come back. You may well be most vehemently reassured by a myriad of well-qualified, articulate and quite plausible professionals that what they are proposing is the best possible option for you and your child, but in reality it is often the only option

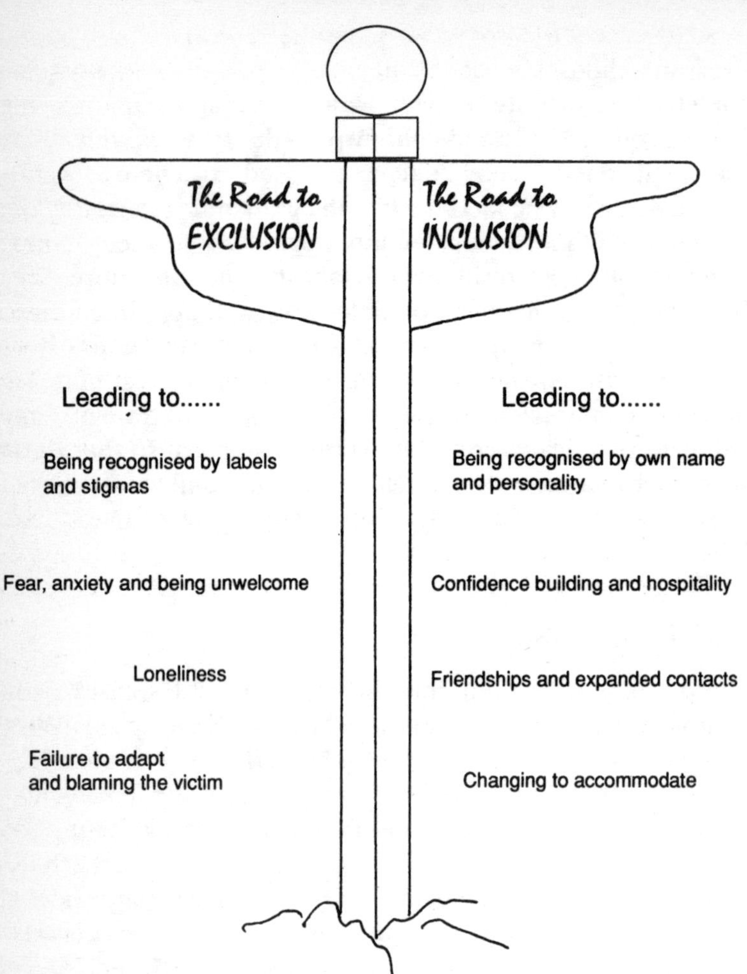

Figure 5. *Choosing the direction to take.*

they have to offer, or perhaps the least expensive for their ever-decreasing budgets; or it may even be the most convenient arrangement for them. So what is this road to EXCLUSION that you should be so worried about, and where does it lead? (See Figure 5.)

BEING RECOGNISED BY LABELS AND STIGMAS

Our traditional systems of caring appear to be born from some sort of herding instinct, since much of the provision that we make seems largely based upon categorising people and placing them all together under one roof. Whole batteries of human services are built around labels which are clinically attached to people. Strangely enough, these labels usually seem to end in the suffix 'ics'—'geriatrics', 'alcoholics', 'epileptics', 'phobics', 'anorexics', 'autistics'. . . We have wards in hospitals for anorexics, homes for geriatrics, special schools for autistics—the very label immediately depersonalises and presents people in a most negative light. It takes a person who is by nature multidimensional and in one quick flip of the tongue reduces him or her to a one-dimensional object. He is a 'special needs' child, they say, emphasising first the label 'special needs' and following on, almost as an afterthought, with the fact that he is also a child.

Labels originated from the medical profession and are merely a form of short-hand which depersonalises people and turns them into 'cases' and 'patients'. Putting someone's fractured leg in a plaster cast is seen as a much simpler procedure by some doctors and nurses when they perceive that person as an object. By calling him a 'patient' or a 'casualty' or a 'road accident victim', they can then treat the fracture as an uncomplicated mechanical process. Once the task has been carried out they can just label the person and send him along to the appropriate department at outpatients, much as we do luggage at airports. In real terms, however, 'patients' have names of their own and lives of their own. From the medical standpoint it may be all right for the doctor to say, 'I'll see the broken leg next.' But of course each broken leg will be attached to a quite different person. It may be the broken leg of someone who is a professional footballer whose livelihood will therefore become severely affected. Even worse, it could be the leg of the mother of five young children in a one-parent family situation.

Whatever the circumstances, each person will have vastly differing needs, and whilst we may have become well practised in attending to one aspect of people's need, we certainly have a long way to go in offering practical and very necessary support for their more fundamental difficulties. Whilst we may be treating symptoms quite well, we really haven't yet discovered how to cure many of the root problems. The plain and simple fact is that labels are for luggage; people, on the other hand, have names. The more people refer to your child by labels rather than his name, the farther down the exclusion road you will be travelling.

FEAR, ANXIETY AND BEING UNWELCOME

Special systems, which segregate people, may in all honesty be designed to address specific needs, but in reality they prevent those who have additional needs from participating, along with the rest of us, in everyday living. Such systems serve to highlight the differences between people. They keep those who are deemed to be below par in some way from living alongside the rest of us. People are made to go to different schools, live in different accommodation and spend their leisure time mostly with each other in special clubs and special institutions, but not in the community at large. It is not surprising, therefore, that they become unknown in their own neighbourhoods and it is not long before fear of this unknown takes its toll. Everyday folk tend to become wary. These people who are kept in different places, we erroneously assume, must be dangerous, a risk to the rest of our society. When we come across them we may well find ourselves treating them with suspicion and caution. Our uneasiness means that we avoid eye contact with them, give them a wide birth, turn our backs on them and discourage their attempts even to pass the time of day with us. Fear and anxiety reign not only with the general public, but with those who are rejected and made to feel unwelcome. After constant rebuffs and coolness from others, they too become anxious and fearful about joining in.

LONELINESS

If human beings really are social animals, then none of us is an island; we all need to spend some time in the company of others. Services which declare themselves to be special limit the opportunities of those who use them to meet and share interests with non-disabled people who live in their locality. Friends, contacts and simple acquaintances are difficult to cultivate if you are largely restricted to meeting only those people who are labelled as having the same type of disability as yourself. The trouble is, our society seems to be caught up in what Judith Snow refers to as 'idolising the average'. It's a vicious circle that we have to break. The more we separate people on the basis of their disability, the more we breed conditioned people who think that it is appropriate to do this. In such a culture, a person who has additional needs is seen as somehow needing to be 'fixed'. It is this attitude, reinforced by special and separate services, that prevents many budding relationships from developing on an equal footing. Equal that is, in the sense of regard that exists. Many 'friendships' are established on the carer or befriender basis, but this is a far cry from what true companionship is all about. If the school that you attend is quite different from the other schools in your area, if it is also stigmatised with the word 'special' appearing somewhere in the title, and if it is situated some miles from where you live, then not only will you have difficulty in meeting other children who live nearby, but when you do, their perception of you (if not one of fear and caution) is likely to be condescendingly overcompensating.

Loneliness is not only about having few people around, it can also be about having many people around but none of whom relates to you as a friend, listens to you or tries to tune in to what you want to communicate, none of whom seems capable of seeing beyond your additional needs to the person who is you. A loving husband and wife can have their relationship transform quite dramatically into one of carer and patient should either one of them contract a condition like multiple sclerosis. Whilst nursing may become an added feature in their lives to deal with specific needs, it is their perception and relationship to one another as a married couple that needs to remain paramount. By the same token, mothers and fathers must establish and maintain their parenthood above all else as their primary relationship with their disabled sons and daughters.

FAILURE TO ADAPT AND BLAMING THE VICTIM

On the whole, those special services that we have developed to date seem to have, woven into their very fibre, an unwritten understanding that those who provide the service must somehow hold status and power over those for whom the service has been designed. Psychologists, therapists, heads of special schools, managers of adult training centres and various bureaucrats have almost total control over what service is provided, how it is provided, where and when it is provided. They quite forget that the only reason their profession exists at all is to serve those people in our communities who have additional needs. This is the only reason why such professionals are able to earn a living and pay their mortgages.

However, much of the time services seem to be geared to the convenience of the provider rather than the user. If you have additional needs, you will of course want to seek out ways in which you can receive this support. The problem is that you are not given any purchasing power with which to buy it; instead, you will have to accept what is on offer, whether it is suitable or not. Contrary to how it should be, it often turns out to be the special services which choose you, as opposed to you choosing them. It is they who decide who comes and goes in their establishments and, what is more, they are not made directly accountable to you for what they do. As a service user, if you complain or in some way express your dissatisfaction and continue to express it, then sooner or later you may well find that blame is apportioned to you for not properly 'fitting in' to the system, or you will be regarded as being unreasonable. Keep pressing your case and you may even find that you are referred to as 'neurotic'. Incredible as it may sound, few special services will change their organisation to meet the needs of those whom they serve. It is you who are expected to adapt to the system of care which they endeavour to make available to you.

Taking the road to inclusion

On the other hand, if you choose to travel down the road to INCLUSION, whilst your journey will still be a little rocky, the outcomes and the destination are likely to be quite different. This is a road which, until now, has been mostly untravelled. As yet there is no map to guide us from A to B, but it is a road which welcomes everyone and by travelling it together we are more likely to overcome any barriers we may come across along the way.

John O'Brien has described three 'monsters' that we are likely to encounter on this road. The first monster we must slay is *Fear*. Our fear of the unknown makes us reluctant to explore a different and unfamiliar path. Most of the time, we will make almost any excuse not to do it—not enough money, poor access problems, not enough staff who are properly trained or experienced. Whatever the reason we give, it is merely an excuse for our own personal fear.

The second 'monster' is a bigger beast and more difficult to overcome. This one goes by the name of *Control*. Whether we are a person with additional needs, a parent or a professional, we have to learn how to share the power of control, so that together we shall be able to plan and carry out better futures for everyone. This means that professionals will have to give up the balance of power which is currently in their favour, in order to work collaboratively with those who use their services—something which most professionals find it difficult to do. They enjoy their position of power over others, their status in the world and their salaries, so they are not likely to give all that up easily. Some parents, too, have to learn to give up the power that they hold over their son or daughter. Parents exercise their power as a measure of protection against their youngster's perceived vulnerabilities. Nevertheless, such control can stifle and cause more harm than good in the long run.

The third 'monster' is *Change*. Although change is constantly going on around us, we seem almost by reflex to want to evade it at all costs. We become extremely inert in order to try and resist that which is inevitable. Change can make us feel most uncomfortable and, like fear, we will often search for any excuse to avoid it. It may well be that there are even more 'monsters' which as yet we know little about, but those who have begun to travel the road to INCLUSION have already reaped some of the benefits.

BEING RECOGNISED BY OWN NAME AND PERSONALITY

When those who have additional needs get the chance to join in everyday local community events as individuals in their own right, as opposed to being taken as part of a disabled group, they soon discover that most other people readily accept them for who they are. They quickly become known by their first names, as opposed to the name of the syndrome with which their condition has been labelled. Consequently, they are assessed more upon their strength of personality than upon their weakness of disability. Ordinary everyday people are more likely to recognise and appreciate skills and giftedness at whatever level, whilst professionals in special services appear to focus more upon a person's lack of skills and inability. Whilst others are seeing you as a person, special services tend to see you as a problem.

There are considerable differences between what you will experience through being a client whose needs are met by a special service and being an included member of your local community. In a community situation, ordinary people will get together and brainstorm your problem in order to come up with a viable solution, whilst in a special service formal meetings and case conferences will be organised, usually at a time and place most suited to the professionals. In the latter a sense of urgency is often absent and a high degree of importance is given to bureaucratic rules. However, when a disabled person is included fully in her community, her friends and acquaintances will often either flout or simply change the rules in order to ensure that her personal needs are met.

CONFIDENCE BUILDING AND HOSPITALITY

Involvement with their local community in ordinary ways means that people with disabilities have the same opportunities to form networks of friends, acquaintances and contacts that the rest of us do. The more people participate, the more they become included and the more they are included, the greater everyone's confidence becomes.

A short time ago, I came across Julie who is now 22 years old. Julie is like most young women of her age and enjoys the company of others, going shopping, pop music and the like. The fact that she has learning difficulties has meant that she has not always been able to express herself as clearly as she would have liked and this has led to considerable frustration on occasions, which in turn has resulted in episodes in which her temper has sometimes got the better of her. Five years ago, the District Health Authority was approached for help. This resulted in Julie being labelled as having challenging behaviour and she was eventually moved from her parents' home and the area she knew well, to a specialist establishment about a hundred miles away.

Five years on this same establishment contacted the Local Authority who were paying the cost of Julie's place there, and informed them that they were no longer prepared to accommodate Julie. The Local Authority decided that they had one of two choices. Either they could place Julie in a similar special unit, or they could spend the same amount of money allocated to her on giving her the chance to live in her own home in the area which she had once known well. Julie chose the latter—a good choice, I'm sure, since over five years the former had proved itself an outright failure.

Over the last few months Julie has been settling in to her new lifestyle. This has not been without incident, of course, but her understanding of how to deal with stressful situations has already grown to such an extent that her adverse behaviour, which still occurs from time to time, is already much less intense and less frequent than it has ever been before. More significantly, she has now developed a circle of some fifty or sixty friends and acquaintances in her immediate locality, with whom she spends time. She visits several of her neighbours and has lunch and tea at their homes; they in turn visit her and have meals with her. She participates in local clubs, catches the bus to go shopping and does all the usual things that other people do.

As time goes by, doubtless Julie will make new friends and lose some of her old friends who may move out of the area. Her network of support and companionship is forever changing and expanding in the same way as everyone else's. She is constantly learning new skills and concepts from the different interests she is discovering and the people she meets. Her special residential placement was a stark contrast to this. Her options there were extremely limited and she had no opportunity in any sense for sustained personal growth. Her new life has meant that the people around her have become confident and hospitable, and so has Julie herself.

FRIENDSHIPS AND EXPANDED CONTACTS

During the course of my travels, I came across a woman who had chosen to take the road to INCLUSION. She told me about her son Steven who was seven years old and had spent the last three years in a special school for children who have severe learning difficulties. At first, like most parents, she had been extremely concerned to learn of her son's additional needs. She had relied heavily upon professional advice and finally placed her child in a special school a good half-hour's drive away from where they lived.

As time passed, she became more and more disillusioned with the special system which seemed to be doing very little to meet Steven's needs. During discussions with the school, she found that although the staff were very pleasant, they were far from encouraging when she asked about the possibility of her son attending his local mainstream school with assistance. Finally she took the bull by the horns and made an appointment to see the head teacher of the school across the road from where they lived, taking Steven with her.

'This is my son,' she said. 'He is seven years old and has lived over the road since he was born. He doesn't have any friends, he doesn't even know any of the children who live around these parts, so he never gets invited to birthday parties or to other people's houses for tea. I wonder if he might just spend one afternoon in the classroom where he would have been if he hadn't been born with a disability.'

It was a request that few head teachers could justifiably refuse. A date was arranged and Steven went along to join in an art class. Almost immediately the other children took a great interest. They asked an inexhaustible tirade of questions. 'What's his name?' 'Can he talk?' 'Why can't he walk?' 'Does he like painting?' 'Can I help him?' There was no standing on ceremony: children became involved straight away and the problem was not one of trying to coax other children into getting to know Steven but more of trying to stem the rush.

By the end of the session the children were anxious to know if Steven would be visiting them again. As a result, a date was set for the following week and the event soon became a regular occurrence. Steven was also invited to share a number of other events with this class in between times. After-school invitations came quite rapidly, and Steven accepted these and also sent out his own invitations to others to come to his home. It wasn't long before the class started to ask some really awkward questions like, 'Why can't Steven come here all the time?' and they refused to be fobbed off with casual answers.

Steven began to go to the school over the road more and more often. Although his mother was pleased, it demanded a great deal of her time if she was always to accompany him, time which she could often ill afford. Anyway, it could hardly be regarded as normal for a child of seven to have his mother with him at school every day.

It was the children who decided to act. They collected no less than two hundred and fifty signatures from all the other pupils; these were attached to a letter addressed to the chief education officer, saying how much they wanted Steven to attend their school all the time and how well he had done from being there up until now. Not only did the chief education officer receive the letter but so did the local press, and the rest is history as far as Steven's mother is concerned. To begin with, an assistant was employed for just two days a week, until it was pointed out that Steven's additional needs were there all the time. It was rather like saying to a blind person, 'Here is a white stick, but you can only use it on Tuesdays and Thursdays.'

Steven no longer attends his special school; he no longer sits at home in the evenings without friends of his own age. He has much wider interests and is now well known in the locality. Opportunities for a fuller life when you take the road to INCLUSION are open-ended.

CHANGING TO ACCOMMODATE

When the fertiliser hits the air-conditioning, whilst many special services seem to be taken up with protecting their own personnel and blaming the victim, inclusive communities are more ready to make adjustments to accommodate the particular needs of an individual who has a disability. In a special service, the individual may be viewed as just another disabled person who has to fit in to the long-established routines and organisation. When that same person becomes part of an ordinary local group, like a school or a club, he or she is often the only person who has a disability and the others tend to pool their ideas and resources, in order to overcome any difficulties.

There is of course a big difference when friends are involved rather than paid professionals, since friends are just as concerned about dealing with your problem as you are yourself. When Clare began to attend her local school instead of the special school she had been attending, it was the other children in her class who decided to use their own resources to design and build a set of portable ramps for her. They had become concerned that Clare couldn't easily manoeuvre her wheelchair into the music class, which they knew she greatly enjoyed. Similarly, in another mainstream school, Michael, who has severe learning difficulties, is never left out of the impromptu football matches that start up at playtimes, because his friends have adapted the rules of their game so that everyone stands still and counts to five each time Michael is in touch with the ball. This way Michael can always join in without making the game unfair for one side. Making small changes to keep people included is important: it means that we can all share and nobody loses out.

In search of guarantees

Whether you decide to take the road to INCLUSION or the road to EXCLUSION, make sure that the choice has been yours. Of course, you will need to listen to what others say to you, but don't let them take away your right to decide. You may be attracted by the benefits that INCLUSION brings, but you may also be put off by that first 'monster' *Fear*. You may want cast-iron guarantees, reassuring you that nothing will ever go wrong. As yet, this cannot be done. We are learning each day about the journey we are taking down the INCLUSION road. Each day, however, the numbers travelling are growing bigger and bigger. The process is beginning to happen in Europe, in America and in Canada and the results are extremely encouraging.

If you are looking for guarantees, then of course, you already have one: what happens if you choose the road to exclusion is very well documented. It will lead your son or daughter to a segregated life, being constantly under-valued and discriminated against, and that is the only guarantee on which you can rely. We know exactly where the road to exclusion leads.

3 Bringing up Baby

> 'The joys of parents are secret and so are their griefs and fears.'
>
> Francis Bacon

All babies, whether disabled or not, are very demanding upon their parents. To start with, they crave their undivided attention for much of the time, require constant supervision and have countless physical needs, most of which seem to centre around food, toileting and general considerations of hygiene. Bringing up a baby necessitates everlasting patience, swift anticipation, understanding and a cool head, and a dozen pairs of hands and eyes, too. Of course few, if any, of us have these attributes in anything like the amount we will need, and so the picture of serenity that is so graphically portrayed by the Madonna and child tends to manifest itself only fleetingly, particularly in the first few months. Much as we love our children (and they do bring a great deal of pleasure into our lives), there can be little doubt that they cause us considerable stress and fatigue, too.

Being there

These days the roles of motherhood and fatherhood are no longer as sharply defined as they used to be. Not so long ago the boundaries were quite clear: where the birth of babies was concerned, fathers were definitely pushed into the background and some, I may say, were secretly glad of it. Now, of course, the whole baby scene has been redefined and fathers are actively encouraged to accompany the mother-to-be to pre-natal classes and to have real involvement on the big day itself.

Nevertheless, there are still some fathers who do not relish the prospect of actually being there and participating in the birth. Whilst they readily accept the wonder and excitement of their baby being born and understand that it is a moving and miraculous process, they do not regard it as a 'spectator sport'. Pressurising such men to attend against their inclination is not always a good idea. Not only does their squeamishness embarrass them, but it may lead to them passing out and becoming just another obstacle for staff to work around, and an additional concern for the mother who is in labour. Some men even feel quite guilty about what they have put their partner through when they witness at first hand the unabridged version of their child's birth passage. A few feel so strongly that, for a while at least, it becomes emotionally impossible for them to get close to their partners and show their affection.

Similarly, there are some women who are not particularly keen for their man to be present at the birth itself, since they are not sure how they themselves are going to react; having the father on the spot simply becomes an added anxiety for them. It may be, too, that they do not want to be seen in what they consider to be some quite undignified positions. Some mothers feel that having their partner visit them after the birth, when they can be seen glowing with maternal radiance as they cradle their baby in their arms, is one thing, but being seen trussed up like a chicken whilst turning red in the face from heaving and straining is quite another. Most women, however, prefer to have the father around to give them confidence and to share in the magic of the whole experience. I'm told that some men become so enthused that they even video the entire procedure from beginning to end. Whom they show it to afterwards is a mystery to me.

Sharing the caring

In these more enlightened times men are expected to become just as involved as women in the day-to-day care of their newly born baby, sharing in all the tasks, with the exception, of course, of breast-feeding. Just like their partners, during the pregnancy expectant fathers build up a picture of perfection in their minds. They may imagine a son who will be handsome, strong and capable and will accomplish all those things in academe, sport or career that they themselves would have liked to achieve, or a daughter who will be pretty and able and will have all the qualities that they believe a woman should have.

When they are told that their baby has a significant disability, the gap between their expectations and the reality is so vast that they go through a grief process, mourning the loss of their idea of a perfect child (see p. 25). Whilst many women will cry quite openly, some men seem to cry inside. Often, their way of dealing with their grief is to put distance between themselves and their child. They tend to leave the everyday chores to their partner and spend longer periods of time with their other children or away from their home altogether. They may start to find reasons for working longer hours at their job, or spending greater amounts of time in recreation, but not very often with their own family. Such men try to bury their emotions by avoiding talking to others about their feelings—not just their partners, but anyone.

Talking to one another about how each of you really feel, your worries, your insecurities and any nagging guilt that you may harbour, is essential if your relationship is successfully to absorb the sudden shock. Your baby's additional needs will only become disabling for your child, yourself and your family if you allow them to. The task of parenting becomes so much easier and enjoyable if the two of you share in the responsibilities and routines. All babies need love, consistency and security. These are provided when parents are open with each other, communicate their true feelings and support each other in times of emotional stress and physical tiredness.

The sudden responsibility for another totally dependent human being takes some getting used to, particularly when it comes in the form of a baby which is so small and delicate. I can remember bringing home Mandy, our first-born, from the maternity hospital. I was frightened to lift her in case she might break. That night, as she lay in her cot at the end of our bed, I found myself checking on her every whimper throughout the night, just to make certain that she was still breathing. Mandy was a perfectly robust and healthy baby, with no disabilities whatsoever, but I was still very much on pins about having the responsibility of a little person who relied entirely upon my wife and myself. How I would have been had Mandy also had some major medical need is something that I can hardly contemplate.

With the coming of our first baby, we all tend to share a little fear and doubt about our ability to cope. Making these feelings known to your partner, and learning how to manage together, strengthens your relationship as a couple and allows you to grow as parents. It is helpful to get the practical routines worked out between you so that you both have a clear understanding of what is expected of you. When you bring a baby back into your home, whether he or she is disabled or not, one thing is sure: your life is going to change considerably. Just making a simple trip to the shops will mean that you have to mobilise enormous amounts of equipment—a pram or push-chair, a supply of fresh nappies, powder, drinks and bottles and so on. Getting through those first few months is like tackling a major assault course.

Not only do you have to change your life routines but your baby has to adjust, too. Babies sleep only when they are tired and cry when they are hungry, cold, frightened or uncomfortable, all of which are likely to coincide precisely with those times that are most inconvenient for you. Much as you love them, at times babies seem to have an innate ability to do or not do things that are calculated to drive you to the limits of your patience. They somehow have a universal knack of knowing exactly when to choose that crucial moment which can turn you from a rational, calm adult who is in complete control, into a raving or gibbering wreck. Trying to pacify a screaming baby in the early hours of the morning after an exhausting day, with yet another exhausting day to look forward to, is only one such scenario that can transform you from Mother Theresa into Ghengis Khan. At times during those first few trying months you may wish that you had never had your baby, may resent him and feel like doing him harm.

In fact, these common reactions are not so much products of your baby's behaviour as evidence of your own sense of inadequacy, your fear of your inability to cope as a parent and your doubts about things ever becoming any better. Just about every parent has these feelings about his or her own baby and by the time he has grown into a toddler they have probably forgotten just how earth-shattering and frustrating those first few months actually were. The trouble is that if we are not careful, we may bury these feelings and not share them with our partners or others close to us. We are too ashamed of admitting to someone that we have feelings of resentment towards our own baby, that we are disappointed about how things have turned out and that we don't really want this baby intruding on our lives any more. We may feel that we shall never be able to cope and that our baby will never be any better than he is now. Times like this are just as real to most other parents, as are the times when their baby does things which makes them very proud and loving. We celebrate the latter by telling all and sundry every detail, to the point of becoming totally boring, and minimise the bad times by simply laughing them off. Share your true feelings with your partner and you will invariably find that he or she has been feeling much the same and is somewhat relieved not to be alone. Telling each other just how you feel enables you to work closer together, to give each other a break from the tiring but enjoyable business of bringing up a baby.

The more help you can get the better. Being a good parent doesn't mean having to sacrifice your social life entirely, or prevent you from regularly delegating some responsibility to others whom you trust. The fact that your baby has a significant disability should not cause you to feel that only you can properly look after him. If you have learned what to do and how to act and what to be aware of, then so can other people. Don't shut them out, both for your sake and your baby's. Whether they are disabled or not, all babies are entirely dependent upon adults, in their early years anyway. The more help you can get, the less tired you will become, and you will have more quality time to give to your baby when you are in a happier and contented frame of mind.

If a baby-sitting circle exists in your locality, don't avoid becoming part of it simply because your child has a disability. If you keep away from groups like this, you will not only be isolating yourself as a family, but you will be sending a clear message that your baby is so different from everyone else's, and so difficult to deal with, that it is better that you are not a part of normal life. Talk openly to other mothers and fathers about your baby's additional needs. Explain to them your child's condition and your hopes and worries. Other parents will want to know, but will likely find it difficult to ask, not knowing if their interest will upset you. The onus is upon you to set the trend, to overcome your and their embarrassment by showing that your baby's disabilities are not a taboo subject. This will give you the chance to be part of the parent scene in your locality and to show that your child is a baby first and foremost and that his disability, no matter how serious it may seem, is only a secondary consideration. Allow others to handle your child, and feed him or her. Some people need to have first-hand experiences to gain their own confidence in discovering all the remarkable similarities to their own baby, rather than assuming that there are only huge differences.

Whilst the child development clinics that you will be asked to attend are useful places to find out more about your baby's additional needs and rate of progress, you will also need to be on your guard to prevent yourself from being sucked into separate special systems. Often it is at these clinics that professionals, sooner or later, begin to offer you help by sending you to special nurseries or playgroups where only disabled children attend. You would do well to resist them politely and use the knowledge and assistance of other mums and dads whose children are not disabled, to help you to gain a place in the same services that they use.

It is as well to realise, too, that whilst your child development clinic can be very helpful to you and your baby, you need not feel that you have to attend every single week, or even monthly, if everything is going well. As your child gets older and you become more confident, your appointments at the clinic and with the specialist (paediatrician or whoever) can become quite a bind and fairly fruitless for you, particularly if you find that you are waiting around for hours on end and gaining little from them. Keep in touch when you need to, rather than because you feel you ought to.

The professionals may consider themselves experts and specialists, but you are the most important person in your child's life; spending day in and day out with your child, with some basic grounding in his or her particular disabilities, you and your partner will soon become the most knowledgeable people about your child's needs. Remember, professionals are there to give advice, not to make all the decisions and take over your lives. Whilst they will have a great deal of knowledge about your child's condition, they will have very little knowledge about your child as an individual.

If you want to know all that there is to know about your child's particular condition, you will need to get your information from a number of places. Relying upon one specialist to tell you everything is not usually enough. If your son or daughter has actually had a diagnosis, then you can get your hands on up-to-date literature from various voluntary bodies. The local library is a good source of information, not only for books on the subject but also for local groups established in your area. The Citizens' Advice Bureau can also be helpful.

Becoming a regular member of your local group can bring its own difficulties, however, since many of them are subscribers to special and separate services. If this is so, you will find that this becomes just another way of sending you and your child down that old familiar road to exclusion. If when you attend meetings, you discover that they are into a great deal of fund-raising through selling stickers and organising fêtes and so on, and are working towards establishing their own separate groups for outings, then you will know to keep at arm's length. The time you spend fund-raising and grumbling to other members about what little help you seem to get could be better spent joining in normal everyday events with your friends and neighbours and their children. This is not just a way of maintaining normality in your own life, but is also building a network of friends, acquaintances and contacts for your child as time goes on.

If your local voluntary group is too special and separatist-minded, there is nothing to stop you from contacting one or two other parents who don't necessarily have a disabled child, for a regular coffee morning or whatever at your house. If you are a member of a church, this can be yet another way of keeping involved with your local community. One mother told me that she took her daughter in her wheelchair to various church activities for some months. She found that few people spoke to her daughter, not only because her daughter's learning difficulties made it difficult for her to communicate and respond well, but also because most of the congregation were uncertain how they should act. The following week she made a simple badge and attached it to her daughter. It said, 'My name is Claire, please talk to me.'

The ice was broken and these days Claire is very much a part of that church.

Recognising your child's gifts

We appear to grow up recognising some people's gifts and being totally blind to other people's. There is no reason for this, other than our own conditioning which seems to make us completely unaware of the wide range of influences and benefits that those who are disabled and others have upon us. The culture that we call INCLUSION recognises that all people have a gift, no matter who they are.

Just recently I watched the Wimbledon Tennis Championships. I was not alone in doing this, in fact, as always, they were seen by millions around the world. Thousands of people in Wimbledon itself spent considerable amounts of money to buy tickets and took time off work, in order to sit around a grass court and watch two players bat a ball backwards and forwards across a net to each other. This they did hour after hour, day after day, sometimes in blistering heat, and always as if their lives depended on it. Finally, two weeks later, a winner was declared. At this point, as always, there was a televised ceremony and a huge sum of money was handed over to the players by a member of the British Royal Family. Tennis in itself has no intrinsic use of course, yet those playing at Wimbledon had been practising and training for several hours each day over a period of years, sacrificing much of their social lives so that they could devote as much time as possible to refining their skills in hitting a ball to and fro.

Exactly the same could be said of just about any sport, football, cricket, rugby or whatever. Although useless in themselves they provide amusement for many people and a good deal of employment for some who might otherwise be without a job. Although the act of kicking a ball around or running faster than anyone else may seem pretty pointless, these activities do require an enormous number of people and a large amount of resources to make them happen. A need is created for umpires, trainers, coaches, security people, grass-cutters, ticket collectors and box office people, to name only a few. We certainly value those who become exponents of these various sports. We pay them considerable sums of money and elevate them to fame and stardom for their skill in manipulating a ball into a hole or into a net.

The giftedness of those who are disabled is not so immediately apparent to us, yet it certainly exists. For example, when Gavin was born, his parents were eventually told that he had brain damage. Naturally enough, they sought ways in which their son's disability could be minimised, and after a while they came across a system devised by Doman and Delacatto which involved intensive support from a large number of people on a daily basis. Throughout the day and every day, Gavin had to have several people at any one time to help him through his course of treatment. His parents had to increase their circle of friends and acquaintances quite considerably in order to keep the process going; they certainly could not have managed on their own. More and more invitations were issued for individuals to become involved, and more and more acceptances were received from all sorts of people of all ages and from all walks of life. They made personal sacrifices to come and ordinary people did some rather extraordinary things. Simply by being a child who had some obvious needs, Gavin had unleashed his giftedness. He had caused the caring side of people to be expressed. He had caused people to develop personal skills and qualities that might otherwise have lain dormant. He had caused his parents to widen their network of friends and he had aroused a social response in his community that had brought together people who, without him, might never have met.

Our quality of life would be so much the poorer if we did not appreciate the giftedness of tennis stars, singers and musicians, actors and entertainers, sports personalities and various celebrities, but we also have to recognise that our world and our lives would be considerably worsened if the benefits of those less obviously gifted were not made available to us either. Whilst being able to jump higher than anyone else is a gift, there is also a giftedness which comes from having no legs at all.

The differences that exist between us all are the keystones for basic possibilities in our lives. We exist because of the difference between male and female. If we only allow ourselves to see them, gifts are present in all forms of diversity, for wherever there is diversity there is an opportunity for us to experience the benefits of something different. If you bother to look for them, it is not difficult to see the gifts that people bring with them from different cultures, different genders, different social classes, different abilities. By just being there, we each make our fundamental gifts available.

I am not particularly religious myself, but I was touched by the story that was told by Father Patrick Mackan in his book, *Reflections on Inclusive Education*. It is about an ageing priest who had always wondered what Heaven and Hell were like. One night, in a dream, he was taken to Hell. Much to his surprise there were no demons prodding and torturing lost souls, no fires or furnaces burning, just a crowd of angry and irritable people sitting round long picnic tables, each with a bowl of food and a ten-foot long wooden spoon. Whilst they were able to get their spoons into the bowls, no matter how much pushing, shoving and elbowing of each other they did, the people simply did not have enough room to turn their enormous spoons round once they were in the bowls, so they were unable to get anything to eat. Tempers flew and the scene that the priest witnessed was one of great frustration and total dissatisfaction.

Then the old priest was taken to Heaven where, again to his surprise, he found exactly the same scene. People were seated round long picnic tables with bowls of food and ten-foot long wooden spoons. Here, however, there was peace and calm, serenity and satisfaction. Each person was using his or her long wooden spoon to feed the others.

In our everyday lives we have the same opportunities to

acknowledge each other's gifts and to make each other's lives more meaningful and fulfilling. It is a gift to be able to help someone else and it is also a gift to be the reason why more able people use their abilities to support their fellow human beings.

Apply the five essential accomplishments

Some time ago John O'Brien introduced the notion of five essential accomplishments that need to be taken into account when considering the prospect of supporting someone who has additional needs. It is as well for parents to understand the relevance of these five accomplishments, so that they can apply them and ensure that they are applied by others from day one in their child's life. These accomplishments are known as:

Community presence
Protection of rights and promotion of personal interests
Competence development
Status improvement
Community participation

Applying these accomplishments, and continually asking yourselves if these apply to what your child is experiencing, will go a long way to keeping your youngster on the right road—the road to INCLUSION.

COMMUNITY PRESENCE

If your son or daughter is ever to be fully involved in his or her own locality, have the opportunity to develop neighbourhood friendships, be included in all the local events and happenings and have all the typical everyday experiences that enable people to see things and behave in the same way as everybody else, then you must make certain that your child remains present right there with all the other children, having broadly the same sort of childhood as they do. It is important for you to ensure that your child, just like other children, always experiences daily life in ordinary everyday local community settings. Resist any attempts by various professionals and their services to direct your son or daughter into separate or special places where he or she will simply gain abnormal experiences and have no chance of leading an ordinary life. The children in your area share the same shops, playgroups, health centre, restaurants, buses, trains and schools. Make sure that your child doesn't have to use different ones. Try to make certain, too, that he or she does not use these same facilities only when taken as a member of a group with several other disabled children. If your son or daughter is to gain any individuality and identity within the neighbourhood, it will certainly not be by being hidden within a group of children with similar disabilities.

PROTECTION OF RIGHTS AND PROMOTION OF PERSONAL INTERESTS

Make every effort to act as an advocate for your child's best interests. Don't allow yourselves to be easily overshadowed by professionals or anyone else, simply because you assume, or they encourage you to believe, that they are in some way superior or know better than you. In all that you do, try your level best to ensure that your child has the opportunity to communicate his own feelings in the matter, express his interests and learn to exercise as much informed choice as he can. When it comes to making decisions for your growing child, don't just see things from your own point of view; you will probably only see your own anxieties if you do. Try to see things from your child's standpoint. What is he likely to be experiencing? Will this narrow or broaden his everyday opportunities for developing real friendships and leading a meaningful life?

COMPETENCE DEVELOPMENT

Try to see that your son or daughter has the opportunity to develop a repertoire of personal skills that will be relevant for a meaningful life with others in the community. Your child needs skills which will enable him or her to have real relationships, develop and extend particular personal interests and which can be applied in a natural community environment; avoid skills that only have relevance or use in a segregated institution.

STATUS IMPROVEMENT

It is important to protect your child's persona. Do not allow him or her to be presented to others in such a way as to be considered an object of charity or of pity. Don't dress her or treat her in a way that is much younger than her actual age. Don't let people see her as a medical condition rather than a person, or as someone of whom they should be wary. How others perceive your child will determine how he or she is treated and on that basis opportunities will be opened or closed for her.

COMMUNITY PARTICIPATION

Actively encourage and support your child's natural relationships with others within your family, with neighbours and with his classmates at school. Try to widen his networks of personal relationships with those who are not themselves disabled. Have other children home to play and allow your child to play at his friends' houses. Make sure that you increase, rather than decrease, the opportunities that your child has to maintain and extend his relationships with local non-disabled people. Start when he is young to let go a bit and allow others to help you and share in the responsibility of ensuring that your son or daughter participates in all the usual things in which other children of that age participate.

Enjoying their milestones and avoiding the millstones

In the early years, you are likely to find that many professionals will display an almost pathological interest in how your child is coping with his or her milestones. By this they mean how she is comparing with other children when it comes to achieving a range of competencies in her stages of development. They will be on the look-out for undue lateness in walking, talking and so on. One of the more useful professionals (in the practical sense) whom you are likely to come across from the very beginning is a health visitor. They are usually very good at establishing a sound rapport with mums and dads and are in a good position to help you with some of the everyday things that may be causing you to worry. Health visitors are also good people to know when it comes to discovering what and who else can be of real assistance to you, such as specialists and other professionals who can give you advice and resources. They can put you in touch with relevant voluntary organisations and, better still, other parents who are going through, or have been through, exactly what you are experiencing. However, even health visitors are not exempt from recommending 'special' places to you, so be on your guard against being sent anywhere that caters for disabled children only.

I have never forgotten my first encounter with a health visitor and I don't suppose for one minute that she has either. Our daughter Mandy was a mere eleven days old and we had brought her home from the hospital just a day before the health visitor knocked on the door. She stood in the doorway, wearing a dark blue mackintosh, carrying an ominous-looking bag and sporting a knowing but reassuring grin. I have to say that her timing was spot on and I was extremely glad to see her. I was in the middle of changing a nappy for the first time in my life and had left Mandy sprawled across the bed, half-done.

'Am I pleased to see you,' I said with great relief, and led her to where the action was.

'Carry on,' she said, 'don't mind me,' and she watched as I made a proverbial pig's ear of folding a nappy into a shape that was supposed to resemble a kite. Wisely, she made no attempt to take it all out of my hands—after all, how was I to learn if she simply did it for me? With patience and whilst stifling a grin, she continued to give me verbal instructions until I finally got the hang of it.

'And where's your wife?' she asked.

'She's in the bedroom lying down for a few minutes, she has a headache,' I explained.

'Well, if she had had a headache nine months ago, you wouldn't have to be changing nappies, would you?' she said with a nudge of her elbow and a wry-looking smile. I knew that I was going to like this woman. Mandy had been breast-fed in hospital, but this was quite beyond my capabilities even as one of society's 'new men', and I proceeded to get a bottle ready.

'What are you doing about sterilising?' the health visitor asked, which took me by surprise. I turned to her a little nervously.

'Well, actually, we want to have more children,' I said, provoking a squeak of laughter.

'No no no,' she giggled, nodding her head towards the Milton equipment. 'I mean the baby's bottle.'

Whilst the development of babies follows pretty much the same pattern in terms of the order that is followed, the rate at which each infant progresses will be quite different. Children will learn to walk before they can run and reach for an object before they can pick it up, but how quickly they are able to move from walking to running, or from reaching to grasping, will vary considerably, even where there is no disability present. The following is designed to give parents a rough guide to some of the things professionals look for in the examinations at baby clinics, in developmental terms, from one month to two years. I do not propose to go into great detail, since there are already several books published on this topic, which are easily available. For those interested I would recommend *From Birth To Five Years—Children's Developmental Progress* written by Dr Mary Sheridan and published by NFER-Nelson.

ONE MONTH

Physical

Will display large jerking movements of arms and legs with arms being more active.

When they are at rest, their hands are closed with thumb turned in.

Their fingers and toes will fan out with big arm and leg movements.

When held in a sitting position their back appears as one curve.

When the corner of their mouth is touched they will turn their head towards it and try to suck.

When they are held in a standing position on a hard surface, they will show a walking movement.

Sight

Their pupils react to light.

They will turn their head towards sudden light.

They follow a pen torchlight with their eyes at a distance of twelve inches.

Will shut their eyes tightly when a light shines straight into their face.

Will hold a gaze at objects that are dangled in front of them across their field of vision.

Watch adult's face intently sometimes when being fed.

Hearing and speech

Are startled by sudden noises.

Cry with some gusto when hungry or uncomfortable.

Sometimes make gurgling sounds when they are content.

Their whimpering can sometimes be stopped by talking to them.

Social development

Have a good sucking action.

Coo sometimes.

Will sleep much of the time, when not being fed.

THREE MONTHS

Physical

Kick legs vigorously at times.

When pulled to a sitting position, they don't let their head lag.

Hands are held open more.

When held in the sitting position, their back is straighter, except at the bottom part of their spine.

When put onto their front, they hold up their head and upper chest.

When held in a standing position on a hard surface, legs tend to sag at the knees.

Sight

Will now become very interested in faces that are close to their face.

Will turn their head to look around.

Sometimes watch people who pass by.

Look at their own hands in front of their face and play with them.

Get excited at seeing their bottle produced when they are hungry.

Have a clear defence blinking action.

Hearing and speech

Sometimes smile at the sound of a familiar voice.

Respond with vocal sounds sometimes when spoken to.

Sometimes make gestures like smacking lips together as food is being prepared.

Can get excited when hearing sounds like someone approaching, or bath water running.

Social development

Look intently and contentedly at adult when being fed.

Show enjoyment of various routines like bathing, etc.

Enjoy games with sounds, faces, tickling, etc.

SIX MONTHS

Physical

When laid on their back they sometimes grab hold of their own foot.

Sit with some support and turn head around to look at different things.

Kick very strongly sometimes with alternating legs.

Will roll over front to back and back to front.

Keep head firm when held in a sitting position.

Can bear their own weight with their legs when supported on a hard surface.

Sight

Look everywhere eagerly.

Watch various people with great interest.

Eyes move together in unison.

Use whole hand to grasp things with.

Pass toys, etc., from hand to hand.

Follow things like balls that are rolled past them, if interested enough.

Hearing and speech

Know the voices of familiar adults.

They practise their own vocal sounds.

Laugh, chuckle, scream, etc.

Start to recognise different emotional tones in an adult's voice.

Social development

Reach for and grasp hold of nearby toys, etc.

Put most objects to their mouth.

Will take a rattle when offered and attempt to shake it.

Look very closely at objects as they pass it from one hand to the other.

Can sometimes show signs of shyness with strangers.

NINE MONTHS

Physical

Will sit unaided for up to ten or fifteen minutes.

Keep balance better when leaning across to pick something up.

Can turn body sideways to reach for things.

May try to crawl.

Whole body and limbs can be very active sometimes when in their cot or pram.

Try to pull themselves into a standing position.

When held in a standing position, they will attempt a walking action.

Sight

Manipulate toys and objects with a lively interest.

Begin to use index finger to prod things and to point.

Sometimes get hold of string between finger and thumb to pull a toy.

Sometimes watch the path of a marble rolled past them at a distance of ten feet.

Show a good visual interest in the things going on around them.

Hearing and speech

Listen attentively to everyday sounds.

Often make verbal sounds as an attempt to make their thoughts and feelings known.

Will imitate sounds made by adults in a game.

Babble loudly at times.

Sometimes shout to get your attention.

Begin to understand 'no' and 'bye-bye'.

Social development

Hold, bite and chew a biscuit.

Bring their hands around a cup or bottle when drinking.

Have a good idea of the difference between strangers and familiar people.

Still put everything to their mouth.

Copy hand-clapping and enjoy a game of peek-a-boo.

Can find a toy that is half-hidden under a cushion if interested.

Sometimes try to get hold of the spoon when being fed.

ONE YEAR

Physical

Can sit up well, unsupported, for quite a long time.

Can get themselves into a sitting position from lying down.

May well be crawling in some fashion.

Will pull themselves up by holding onto furniture and let themselves down again.

Try to walk around furniture by holding onto it.

Walk forward or sideways if their hands are held.

Sight

Pick up small sweets and other objects using finger and thumb.

Throw toys and watch them fall.

Look in the right place for toys that are out of sight.

Point with index finger to things that they want or interest them.

Start to look at some pictures.

Hearing and speech

They recognise their own name when called.

Make sounds which incorporate most vowels and consonants.

They understand some of what is said to them, particularly when gestures are used.

May give an adult things for which they are asked.

Social development

Will drink from a cup with only a little help.

Can fairly quickly find a toy that is hidden in front of them.

Play 'pat-a-cake' and wave 'bye-bye'.

Drool less.

Help with dressing by doing things like holding arms out, etc.

Like to have a familiar adult within sight.

Like and play with toys that make sounds.

FIFTEEN MONTHS

Physical

Starting to make serious efforts to walk but very unsteadily.

Beginning to try and walk upstairs.

Will sometimes kneel with only a little help.

Sight

Quite precise with both hands in picking up string or small objects with finger and thumb.

Will put one toy brick on top of another.

Will hold a large crayon with whole hand and attempt to make a mark.

Look at brightly coloured books with interest.

Hearing and speech

Will make lots of jabbering-type sounds.

May be able to use up to around six familiar words properly.

Point a good deal at familiar people and things and use vocal noises in support.

Understand and obey simple vocal requests.

Social development

Start to hold spoon when eating.

Help more constructively when being dressed.

Rarely put toys into mouth.

Show a good deal of interest in things and people around them.

They are in exploration mode and need an eye kept on them constantly.

Will push along a large wheeled toy.

EIGHTEEN MONTHS

Physical

Beginning to walk more steadily.
Begin to try running.
Pull and push large toys around the room.
Can kneel upright without any support.
Will climb into a big chair and turn round in it to sit.
Will often carry a large doll or teddy whilst walking.
Will try to walk upstairs if given a good deal of help.
Will sometimes squat to pick up something.

Sight

Can hold a narrow pencil in some way and attempt to use it.
Will scribble to and fro.
Can build a tower of around three toy bricks.
Enjoy simple picture books and turn pages, several at a time.

Hearing and speech

They will jabber to themselves whilst playing.
Will be saying anywhere from 6 to 20+ words and will understand a lot more.
Will enjoy nursery rhymes and may try to join in.
May try to sing.
Will carry out simple requests like 'Get Mummy's shoe.'

Social development

Will feed themselves and chew well.
Can drink by holding a cup with both hands.
Will sometimes take off socks and shoes.
Will still be wetting themselves but will call for the toilet.
They may have some bowel control if you are very lucky but this is very variable.
Will play by putting things in and out of containers.
Will not now be putting toys into their mouth.
Sometimes very clingy, sometimes very independent.

TWO YEARS

Physical

Run with confidence and a certain amount of dexterity.
Will squat without overbalancing.
Can throw a small ball without falling over.
Can walk backwards pulling a toy.
May walk upstairs carefully by holding onto a banister.
Will likely walk into a large ball whilst trying to kick it.

Sight

Can take the wrapping off a small sweet.
Will turn the pages of a book singly.
Will hold a pencil like an adult.
Have usually established a preference for their left or right hand.
Will recognise familiar adults from photographs but not themselves.
Will scribble in a circular motion.

Hearing and speech

Will likely be using about fifty or so words and will understand a lot more.
Listen more to people.
Will be able to link two or more words together to make a simple phrase or sentence.
Will say the names of things from pictures.
Will repeat over and over again some things that people say.
Will talk to themselves a great deal.

Social development

Will spoon-feed themselves quite well.
Will ask for food or drinks.
May become jealous of attention shown to other children.
Usually will be mostly dry throughout the daytime.
Can be very resistant and rebellious at times.
Frustration may well lead to tantrums.
Will play next to other children but not really with them.

Will defend their own possessions.
Will demand attention all the time and drive you nuts.
Will tell you that they need the toilet, usually in time.

* * *

In the early days, parents of disabled children quite naturally feel vulnerable. They are having to cope with the shock of discovering that their child is not going to be as they expected. They are very unsure about the full consequences of this and even more unsure about precisely what their son's or daughter's needs are and how they should be meeting those needs. There is a temptation to rely heavily upon the specialists and even to relinquish parental responsibility to 'those who know best'.

Allow the news of your child's disability to bring you and your partner even closer together. Talk to each other and support each other, not only in the daily physical routines but on the course you intend to take in your child's upbringing. Avoid making ordinary things special and invite others around you to participate in your child's life. Don't try to do it all on your own.

4 Schooling—the Best Years of Their Lives

'Don't major in minor things.' H. Jackson Brown, Jnr.

What is education for?

Oddly enough, it appears to be educationalists themselves who, more often than not, take a fairly narrow view of what education is really all about. Much of their focus of attention seems to become concentrated almost entirely upon the academic attainment of children. I suppose most of us are the same. When we think about our children's education, what immediately spring to mind are the academic subjects and how well they are doing in them. We hope or expect our children to achieve certain standards, particularly in subjects like mathematics and the Queen's English. Reading, writing and arithmetic become those all-important subjects which we refer to, somewhat paradoxically I always feel, as the 'Three R's'. These we hold in the highest esteem and some of us can become quite anxious if we feel our child is not achieving the grades or standard attained by others in his class.

It is drummed into us from our own school days that, unless you pass the dreaded exams in these key subjects and demonstrate your mastery of them under test conditions, then you will not gain for yourself the advantages in adult life of securing a 'good' job and a comfortable way of living. The trouble is that we often seem to view education with tunnel vision. It is as though we have binoculars permanently welded to our eyes, so that all we focus upon and magnify is children's adeptness in dealing with words and numbers, which is of course important but only part of the picture. In a world where we have so many breakdowns of communication, conflicts, violence, crime and insurrection, surely the ability to relate well to others, to understand the need for and abide by a sound moral code of behaviour, and to have developed an awareness and concern for others, are just a few things which must be equally as important as the ABC. It is interesting to discover that a few years ago a large corporation carried out a survey to find what factors made employees successful in their jobs. Fifteen per cent turned out to be related to qualifications, but an enormous 85 per cent were simply people skills.

As I write, I can't help being reminded of George, who used to live in the East End of London. In his formative years, George had found schooling pretty boring and, what's more, he felt that it cut severely into his day, preventing him from doing those things which he thought much more interesting. As a result, George's attendance in class was pretty minimal. Most of the time he 'wagged it'.

Not surprisingly, George left school without the benefit of being able to read or write. In fact he was not even able to sign his own name. But like most people who are illiterate, George had learned to cover his tracks well and became quite skilled in hiding his unfamiliarity with the written word. For a number of years he was employed by the Local Council as a public convenience attendant and he did the job rather well. He took great pride in his work. People regularly commented upon the standards of hygiene that George maintained and the way he carried out his duties with a beaming smile for everyone and a witty sense of humour that added to their day.

As time passed, the Local Authority changed their system of ordering fresh stocks of soap, paper tissue, disinfectant and so on. George was suddenly expected to complete order forms on a weekly basis. Try as he might, he was finally unable to hide his secret and, despite his success in the job for so long, bureaucracy got the better of him and he had to leave.

George had to earn a crust somehow, and sooner rather than later. He used all his resourcefulness to begin his own window-cleaning round. His cheerful personality and ability to work hard meant that he went from success to success. His first window-cleaning round grew to such an extent that he had to take on another worker, then another and another, until he had developed several very successful rounds.

George became financially quite comfortable and his cheeky repartee endeared him to many people, which meant that he gained, over time, a wide circle of friends. One night he was holding a party at his home and, running short of drinks, he went into his bedroom, reached below his bed and pulled out a suitcase full of cash. His friends were horrified.

'What if you are burgled or the house burns down? You'll lose everything. Why don't you keep it in the bank, for God's sake?'

The answer of course was simple. George found form-filling and the idea of cheques quite impossible. The next morning a few of his friends went along with him to the bank and explained the situation to the manager. In opening his account, George proceeded to hand over the notes in the suitcase. The bank manager sat back aghast.

'If you can earn all this money without being able to read or write,' he said, 'think where you would be now if you could.'

'I know exactly where I'd be,' said George. 'I'd be a toilet attendant for the Council!'

We need to ask ourselves why we are educating our children—for what? Academic skills are important, of course, and each child should have the opportunity to achieve as much as he or she can, but it really shouldn't become our only consideration. More than anything, we ought to be educating our children to become good citizens for the future, and for that they need to have a sound sense of morality, a social conscience and an ability to develop good relationships. They need to learn how to value and respect each other, to acquire a caring nature and build a way of life which is beneficial for all. We know that in the late 'thirties and early 'forties it was people who were 'well educated' who committed genocide by gassing, shooting and burning millions of Jews. 'Well educated' doctors inflicted horrendous medical experiments on men and women. Trained nurses poisoned children. So whilst academic achievement is certainly important, educating children to have humanity is essential.

Heads of all educational establishments, from kindergarten to university, should be continually asking themselves, what is it that our students are learning here? Are they developing insight or prejudices? Are they learning to have power over others or power with others? Are they developing a commitment only to their own careers or a commitment to their communities, too? Are they learning values or simply costs? Are they learning how to implement parity or how to mete out charity? Concern for others needs to be a core subject in our curriculum as are English and maths. An educational system which is based upon an attitude that seeks to teach the best and separate the rest, takes away fundamentally from quality learning for all pupils.

Why do we separate children anyway?

Most of us have some idea of what it feels like to be excluded. After all, we are quite likely to have experienced it ourselves from time to time. It may have been because we were too young, or perhaps too old. It may have been because we were of the 'wrong' sex, or because our skin was of the 'wrong' pigmentation. For whatever reason, there will undoubtedly have been those uncomfortable times when we have found ourselves not merely left out, which is bad enough, but deliberately prevented from being included—isolated from the majority into the minority. It is not a pleasant feeling and one which would be difficult for us to sustain over a long period of time without detriment to our confidence, self-esteem, happiness and general well-being.

Knowing how bad it feels, even on a temporary basis, should be enough for us to ask why we would want to impose it permanently upon the people whom we love. Nevertheless, because we are assured by Local Education Authorities that it is for our child's own good, we seem to stand by and watch them go to great lengths, and considerable costs, to identify those children who cannot walk as well, talk as well, or think as well as the average child (if there is such a thing). This is done so that they can exclude these children from the schools that most of our children attend and separate them into 'special' places. They call these places 'special' as though the children who are sent there have been awarded some sort of privilege, an enviable accolade that we all wish we had had bestowed upon us. In reality special schools turn out to be places where children become stigmatised, isolated and unable to experience the same everyday features of life that the rest of us have as a simple matter of course.

Since we ourselves are the products of a segregated education system, most of us, without even realising it, struggle with a deeply ingrained negative attitude towards disability. It is something which we are embarrassed by, uncomfortable with, frightened of, or derisive towards. Equally destructive is the pitying 'Ahhh factor', which is swiftly followed with a phrase like 'poor thing' or 'bless him'. A somewhat innocent or even kind attitude, you may think, until you are on the receiving end of it yourself. Our educational experience of separatism has taught us, in an implicit way, to be fearful of disability because it is unknown to us. We learn that it is different and has to be kept away from our everyday lives, in our schooling, our work and in our leisure time. Disability becomes something that you give money to, do voluntary or charity work with and gradually, over time, the discrimination and prejudices attach themselves in our subconsciousness and grow. We end up saying or thinking things like, 'I've got nothing against disabled people, I think they should be helped, but I wouldn't want my daughter to marry one.'

Excluding those who have a disability from our everyday lives is now such a natural thing for us to do that we no longer see the detrimental effects and severe restrictions it imposes upon the life of a disabled person. Neither do we see how we miss out on the richness in our own lives by not having disability as a natural part of our own daily experience. We have geared the facilities in our communities to meet the needs only of those who can walk, talk, see, hear and have a certain level of understanding. Everyone else has to use different facilities of their own, or simply take their chances.

We have been conditioned to compete rather than to collaborate and have learned that it is important for us to have all the intellectual and physical advantages that we can muster in order to win. However, our win-or-lose way of life means that for every winner there will always be several losers. What we desperately need to implement is a win/win system, in which we all contribute to each other's success. At the moment, our education system is riddled with ways in which we are subtly wooed into striving against one another as opposed to learning how to work together. Musical chairs, for example, is designed in such a way that, when the music stops, there are fewer chairs than there are competitors. As a result, young children learn to push and shove until they get themselves seated at the expense of someone who is not as quick or assertive. How simple it would be, and how much more productive, if instead of leaving one chair for children to fight over, they were rewarded for seeing how they could support each other and help everyone to find a place on that remaining chair.

In the distant past, in numerous civilisations, it was the custom to destroy those who were seen to have a disability. There was not only a bias towards the survival of the fittest, but disability was seen as a 'watering down' or weakening of the race. Disability itself has been, and continues to be, the victim of a whole catalogue of misunderstanding. It has been interpreted as the results of evil powers, and epilepsy in particular for a long time carried the stigma that the person was in some way possessed by devils. For years we blamed disability for moral and social degeneracy and it is not so very long ago that those who were considered to be intellectually disabled were cited as the main reason for criminal behaviour. Superstitions and religious bigotry have also taken their toll and many disabled people were hung or burned as witches. In the Middle Ages, physically and intellectually disabled people were regarded as the 'village idiots' and as such were the butt of ridicule from the other members of the community. It may be that this is how court jesters came into being, and the clowns who are now a traditional part of circuses.

So, in one way or another, if those who had a disability were not killed, then they certainly had some form of isolation forced upon them. In the past this was done with the use of asylums or workhouses and other similar institutions. Nowadays, particularly in educational settings, segregation continues to operate in much the same way as it has always done. The names of the institutions have been changed and perhaps sound more acceptable, but in essence much remains unaltered. Special schools and special units, special clubs for those who are disabled, Adult Training Centres and residential homes, all continue to keep those who are regarded as having additional needs apart from those of us who don't.

More confusingly these days, because care in the community is greatly sought but, sadly, little understood, there are institutions which are in fact no different from the past but try to present themselves as being community based: they ensure that the word 'community' appears somewhere in their title to show that they are conversant with modern-day thinking. So you will now sometimes come across institutions which call themselves something like 'Residential Home for Autistic Community', but those in residence all have the label 'autistic' and find themselves excluded from real community events pretty much as they have always been. Not much will have changed for them, except perhaps the name of the place where they live.

* * *

We know from the findings of the Warnock Committee (who were the authors of a Government Report on Special Education in 1979) that at any one time 20 per cent of our school population will be in need of some form of special education. Two per cent of our schoolchildren are placed in special schools. In planning educational services for these children, we deliberately choose to exclude them from learning alongside the others. The basis for this reasoning is not always clear. History shows that the reasons for excluding disabled people have been unfounded, illogical, unfair and ill-conceived, but we still persist in doing it. Why? Whereas once we said that those who were disabled brought bad luck, were bedevilled, weakened the nation's stock and were responsible for our moral and social breakdown, now we say that it is for their own good. Children who have special needs, we say, must have these needs met by specially trained staff in specially built schools with special programmes of work. 'When it comes to special education,' one parent told me, 'I think it is neither special nor education.' Whilst the word 'special' implies something extra, in reality it is simply a way of investing in an elitist system, one which identifies children as either making the grade or not. A number of myths have grown up around special schools, false assumptions which, if you are not careful, will be used as arguments to convince you that it is beneficial for your child to be sent to one.

Five myths about special schools (There are plenty more)

MYTH NUMBER ONE: 'SPECIAL SCHOOLS PROVIDE A SAFER ENVIRONMENT

You may well be told, and indeed you may yourself already believe, that your son or daughter will be at too much risk in a mainstream school, but well supervised and looked after in a special school where staff are specially trained. In reality, special schools tend to be more dangerous places for disabled children than mainstream. In a special school your child will simply be one of many who have additional needs. In fact, all the other children in that school will have considerable difficulties, too. There will be children who are regarded as hyperactive and children who have challenging behaviour, or what Herb Lovett refers to as having 'severe reputations'. If your child has difficulties with mobility, or is unable to talk or make herself easily understood, then sharing facilities day after day with other children who are perhaps unpredictable and excessively boisterous is, whatever way you look at it, a risky business.

It will be said, of course, that the favourable staffing ratio afforded to special schools ensures that accidents and personal injuries are kept to a minimum. The fact is that all special schools which I have come across are constantly complaining that they do not have enough staff and are continually battling with their Local Education Authority for more personnel. Naturally they will not readily make this known to parents of prospective pupils and will paint the best picture they can of what their school can offer, omitting the areas where they have difficulties and concerns. It does not take a mathematician to work out the problems that special school staff face, when even at the generous ratio of, say, one teacher to seven children (all with severe learning difficulties), close supervision of individuals becomes rather impossible. Even where a classroom assistant is made available, it only takes one child to be assisted with toileting to reduce the staff in the class by 50 per cent.

Conversely, in a mainstream school, there will be perhaps twenty-five or thirty other pupils in the class who between them and their teacher (and perhaps a classroom assistant with knowledge of your child's particular needs) will have just one child with additional needs to support. They, of course, will be in a much stronger position to see that your child comes to no harm. Whilst friends in a mainstream school have the ability to help, classmates in a special school cannot.

When Amy attended her special school, her epilepsy caused her to fall a great deal and she often damaged herself, sometimes quite nastily. Throughout one school term alone, she was taken to the hospital casualty department no less than five times to receive stitching to her head and face. In her class of eight children, one teacher and one assistant, there was not enough staff to prevent these accidents, as there were two other children there who had equal difficulties with their epilepsy and two more who regularly lost their tempers and threw things. At playtime, the situation was worse, since just two staff were on duty for four classes of disabled children, in order that other staff could take a break. Lunchtimes were the most dangerous of all, since they lasted for an hour with minimal staffing supervision.

Amy transferred to her local mainstream school three years ago and, despite the continuance of her epilepsy, has sustained no further injuries. Her class is full of willing friends who between them are on a constant look-out for her welfare in all that she does. Even Amy's school doctor has found that she has more time available for Amy. When she visited her once a year in the special school, time was always fairly limited since all the other children the doctor had to see also had complex medical conditions. In the mainstream school, however, which the doctor also visited annually, very few children are medically anything other than A1, which means that she can spend longer considering Amy's medication and other specific health needs.

'But what about the bullying and jeering that goes on in mainstream schools?' parents ask. In my experience, I have not known anything but care and concern shown by the other children who, once they are made aware of their new classmate's needs, not only seem to become very involved but also become extremely creative in finding ways of overcoming any difficulties that may arise. Recently a group of ten-year-olds were asked to attend a conference so that they could tell the adults there what it was like to have someone in their class (Claire) who had considerable physical and learning difficulties. In her early years Claire had been in attendance at two special schools for children who have severe learning difficulties. She is unable to walk, has to use a wheelchair and cannot speak, and had her parents not created the opportunity for her to attend her local school full time, then she would undoubtedly still be in a special care unit. At the conference, Claire's friends could hardly understand what all the fuss was about. To them Claire was simply a part of their lives, like other children. Their teacher asked them to write down their feelings about Claire and here's what they wrote:

When Claire first came to our school, we didn't know how to communicate with her, but after a while, we all knew. I meet Claire outside school at Church and Drama.

David

Claire teaches us that we all need friends to count on. We are all special, we help each other. Claire lives near me. We enjoy listening to music together.

Bernadette

Claire needs friends like all of us. She helps us to learn about disabled people. Claire is a big part of our community. I am happy when she is nearby.

Danie

I go out with Claire in the holidays. She supports my football team. Claire has changed my life.

Richard

Claire comes to my house for tea. I talk to her when something's wrong. She cheers me up. She is a good friend.

David

We have learned that all handicapped children are important. If Claire can join in our activities then other handicapped children can too. I have invited Claire to my birthday party.

Anna

MYTH NUMBER TWO: 'SPECIAL SCHOOLS HAVE SPECIAL FACILITIES'

Unlike mainstream schools, special schools, we are told, are designed specifically for disabled children. Well, some are and some are not. For years, there was in the North of England a school for children who have severe learning difficulties, which was in fact an old Victorian house. Children who were unable to walk had to negotiate two long flights of stairs before they could reach a toilet. The front door opened straight onto a busy road. Most mainstream schools would be horrified if they had to cope with these conditions, but a special school had managed day in and day out for several years. When the school was finally closed and it was suggested that the children might be better off if they were given support to attend their local mainstream establishments, officers of the Authority asked how they could possibly manage in such schools which would have all sorts of access difficulties.

Whilst this particular special school will not be the only one like this in existence, it is fair to say that most nowadays are at least on one level, and many can be regarded as purpose-built—though for what purpose I am sometimes unsure. Look closely at any special school and note down any significant differences it has from the local mainstream school. Certainly, when it comes to nursery and primary schools, you will be likely to find no great contrasts. There will be classrooms in much the same way as other schools, a staff room, a head's office, an assembly hall that doubles as a dining-room at lunch-time, a playground and all the other facilities that you would expect to find in mainstream education. Perhaps there will be a few more ramps and hand bars around the school, but these are features which can be added relatively easily in most primary schools. If not, then I have to ask how disabled parents get on when they visit their child's school on open day. How does the Council apply its equal opportunity policy for disabled teachers who are seeking to apply for a post in the school? A good many of the problems that are voiced about access in mainstream schools could be overcome with a little thought and goodwill. I often think it would be interesting if our Queen were a wheelchair user. I'm certain that not many of the buildings she was due to visit would declare themselves inaccessible.

Most of Judith Snow's body is paralysed. She has some movement in her right thumb with which she controls the manoeuvring of her wheelchair. A couple of years back she went canoeing. This year she was talking about doing a bungee jump. It's people like Judith who put the difficulties of access in better perspective for those of us who are able-bodied.

One big difference between attending a mainstream school and a special school is that your child will probably be expected to travel miles away from home to get there. This means that some very young and severely disabled children will be taking over an hour to reach their designated special school and over an hour to get home again. This is not something which we would ask of other young children. Instead of gaining the daily experience of crossing roads, meeting other local children along the way, becoming gradually more familiar with their neighbourhood geography, learning the dangers of traffic and so on, your child will more likely be transported on a minibus or taxi into another locality altogether.

Not only does this whole process affect the children themselves, it means that parents, too, can easily become more isolated as a family. Regular interaction with other local parents who congregate twice a day at the school gates, delivering and collecting their sons and daughters, simply does not happen.

Whilst most other parents are seeing their child to school, you will remain at home, on your doorstep, watching your son or daughter be seated in a minibus or taxi.

As well as being quite counterproductive educationally, the cost of ferrying children to and from special schools outside the area where they live is enormous. It is in fact the highest expenditure of any special education budget, with the exception of staff salaries. This money could be used more effectively to offset the cost of engaging a full- or part-time classroom assistant to support your child in his or her local school, as was done in Stockport.

Some special schools will take great pride in pointing out the various special rooms that they may have. The Dark Room or the Light Room or the Light Stimulation Room—it has many names. But whatever it is called it will be a place in the school which is even more isolated and filled with an abundance of flashing coloured lights, soft background music and a whiff of some scent or other in the air. This facility is called 'snoezelen' and over the past few years has started to become the 'in' thing in some special education circles. Head teachers will point to it and announce that they don't have these in mainstream schools.

Setting up a room like this is by no means cheap; it is likely to cost several thousands of pounds. What precisely it achieves, other than a healthy bank balance for the suppliers and a talking point for the school, is frankly quite beyond me and indeed a lot of other people, too. This carefully designed attack on the senses is somehow supposed to stimulate children who they say would otherwise do very little. The fact is that most children respond better to people and are far better stimulated by the company of another person, rather than being subjected to close encounters of the sensory kind. Nevertheless, all kinds of staff seem to spend long periods of time watching and carefully noting down a child's reaction to a moving green or red light. What do they expect to learn from it that will be so beneficial in that child's life? 'Ah,' they say, 'but it can also be used to calm down children who have terrible temper tantrums and rush about throwing things.' In that case, I say, give it to the parents, they are the ones who will need it most.

Another proud feature of some special schools is the fact they have their very own swimming pool. A most laudable measure, I'm sure. However, this only serves to act as yet another way of preventing children who have additional needs from participating in public places alongside their contemporaries. Learning how to swim is of course most important, but much better done in the place where everyone else learns to swim. Exactly the same applies to horse-riding and horse-riding for the disabled. Why do we need to make them separate?

Finally, it is always the toilets that are singled out as being of significant importance in the design of the special school. But what can be so special about toilets that we have to house them in a special school? After all, urine and excrement are pretty universal; disabled children don't produce different forms of them. They don't even produce more than anyone else, although you would be forgiven for thinking so when you see how much time in a special school day is devoted to this function. It is only what goes in that can come out, whoever you are. At most, toilets in a special school can only be used for something like twenty-five hours a week, since that is how long schools are open. And, of course, they are closed for about three months of the year, so what do children do then without these special toilets? Most don't have them at home. Suitable toilets are not so difficult to come by. If shopping precincts, sports centres and swimming pools can have them, it is not beyond our ability to ensure that mainstream schools have them, too.

MYTH NUMBER THREE: 'CHILDREN LEARN BETTER IN SPECIAL SCHOOLS'

There is nothing that is taught in a special school that cannot be taught in a mainstream school. In fact, real learning is more likely to take place in the real world than it is in specially closeted buildings. For one thing, if the other children in your class are unable to speak very well, how are you supposed to learn yourself, without having the benefit of hearing normal speech and language? Odd mannerisms and unsociable behaviour are more likely to be the models that you will experience if the children in your school all have significant learning difficulties.

In talking to various education officers, psychologists and teachers, you may well find that you are left with the impression that mainstream schools are entirely ignorant when it comes to pupils who have special needs and that these needs will be met in their entirety once your child attends a special school. In actual fact, on a national basis, mainstream schools have made a significant investment in staff to address the requirements of such pupils. Most schools now have a written policy which their staff have discussed and are implementing. Additionally, many primary schools have appointed teachers who have a post of responsibility for children who have special needs. Similarly, secondary schools are likely to have a special needs co-ordinator. This has been the case now for the past few years.

As far as special schools are concerned, it is interesting to note the views of the Audit Commission and Her Majesty's Inspectorate, published in the document *Getting In On The Act: Provision for Pupils with Special Educational Needs—The National Picture*. They say: 'The assumption is that once a child is placed in a special school, all needs will automatically be met. This is a mistaken assumption.' They continue: 'Since the passing of the 1981 Education Act, a greater proportion of pupils with special needs is educated in ordinary schools; there is now a high level of awareness of special needs among ordinary school teachers.'

The following extracts from the same document may also prove enlightening:

> It is significant that the quality of the learning experience for pupils with special needs is virtually the same

in both special and ordinary schools, when it might be expected that the presumed higher level of expertise in special schools would lead to a better quality of learning experience for the pupils. The quality of pupil's learning in special schools was affected by a lack of pace in lessons. In addition there was a general absence of assessment and associated response to pupil's individual needs and in some classes a low level of expectation for pupils. This picture is confirmed by HMI reports on the quality of provision in special schools . . .

In too many special schools, the quality of education does not support their becoming centres of excellence for pupils with special educational needs . . .

In 11 out of 12 LEAs, the Chief Educational Psychologist reported that there were pupils in the LEA's special schools who could reasonably be educated in an ordinary school . . .

A number of ordinary school head teachers who said that they had been trying to take on more pupils with special needs, claimed that special schools were over-protective . . .

Most parents of children in special schools who wanted to change, preferred an ordinary school for their child . . .

Most ordinary schools saw themselves as serving the whole local community. Twenty per cent of them saw a positive advantage to their image in taking pupils with special needs, as most head teachers thought that parents were interested in the school's flexibility in meeting individual's needs as well as the overall examination results. This attitude was broadly replicated in the survey of school governors.

MYTH NUMBER FOUR: 'SPECIAL EDUCATION IS CHEAPER'

Finding out the real costs of providing a special segregated education system is not easy to accomplish. Most Local

Education Authorities themselves are unclear what the full costs amount to precisely. Not only do the staffing and transport costs have to be accounted for, but a whole list of other expenditures, such as lighting and heating, stationery and telephone costs, capitation allowances, building maintenance, staff training, and all the additional expense involved in servicing the school from other departments and support systems—personnel back-up, advisory support and the like. The running costs of a whole school are considerable and if we were to calculate the total expenditure it is not unreasonable to expect it to be around £25,000 each year for each child in attendance.

In a special school situation most of this sum is not spent directly on meeting the individual needs of its pupils. A good deal of the costs are lost to items which have little educational relevance to the child and are simply a matter of maintaining the premises. Following their survey into costs, Her Majesty's Inspectorate together with the Audit Commission have written, 'On average it is not more expensive to educate a child with learning difficulties in an ordinary school with support rather than in a special school for pupils with moderate learning difficulties.' Her Majesty's Inspectorate, which is an independent body of experienced educationalists, go on to point out that special school costs have risen significantly in the past five years, since more children who have special educational needs are being educated in mainstream education and fewer are in attendance in the special sector. However, although the special schools have smaller numbers on roll, the staffing resource has remained the same. They therefore estimate that, nationally, around £53 million could have been relocated to support children in mainstream schools in the year 1990-91 alone. Local Education Authorities say that they are reluctant to make this money available to mainstream schools for the following reasons:

1 That if they were to allocate such funding to individual mainstream schools, they would have no guarantee that

it would actually be spent specifically on children who have special needs. However, Her Majesty's Inspectorate feel that there is no evidence to bear this out and that it could not be considered a valid reason, as it would not be difficult for them to put into place systems of accountability when making this funding available.

2 That they consider it a more efficient use of resources for them to maintain a central team of specialists who are better trained in providing for children's special needs than most mainstream schools. Despite this, Her Majesty's Inspectorate found that most head teachers and their staff, in mainstream schools that they visited, did not support this view. Indeed, they felt that they could provide the service more inexpensively and more efficiently. On the whole, they complained that central specialist teams lost much of their time in travelling and often arrived at times which were inappropriate or inconvenient. In addition to this, staff in the mainstream schools got to know individual children much better and related to them more effectively than visiting support staff.

Whilst Local Education Authorities continue to maintain separate special schools, the cost of providing individually supported places in mainstream schools remains an expensive option. On the other hand, closure of a complete special school in order to redeploy each individual child into his or her local school with support, makes the prospect not only viable but more efficient for all concerned.

MYTH NUMBER FIVE: 'CHILDREN GET MORE INDIVIDUAL ATTENTION IN A SPECIAL SCHOOL'

Perhaps one of the greatest myths about special schools is that a child will receive individual attention. On the face of it that appears to be true, and in broad terms it is true. However, you may find head teachers reluctant to say just how frequent this individual attention is. As a visiting parent, it is best not to listen to the sales pitch or the rhetoric, but simply ask to spend the morning or afternoon sitting in the class which your son or daughter would attend. See for yourself just how much time the class teacher is able to give to individual tuition and how relevant that tuition seems to be for the child receiving it. Any good school will be able to show you records of individual programmes of work, but how regularly are these completed and how long does each session last?

With the best will in the world, most teachers in a special school are bound to find it difficult, if not impossible, to provide all the children in their class, on a daily basis, with individual attention that will meet all their needs. This by no means reflects on the teachers' professional ability, it is simply that the special school system prevents them from being as effective as they could be. In medical terms, it is rather like asking the doctor not only to give a prognosis, prescribe medicine and allocate a course of treatment, but expecting him to sterilise the needles, change the beds and give blanket baths, too.

We need the expertise and experience of specialist teachers on a consultative basis, so that their skills can be disseminated and passed over to others who have close and regular contact with the child. The same applies to paramedical staff. These people are so precious and limited in availability that we need them to spread their expertise and empower others with the ability to carry out meaningful day-to-day routines that will benefit the youngster in need. Passing on their skills to parents, classroom assistants and other support staff, who can do the hands-on work on a daily basis, is one of the most beneficial services that an experienced and able professional can perform.

What does the law say?

Before 1971, children whom we referred to as 'mentally handicapped' or 'severely subnormal' were regarded as quite ineducable. Most of them simply remained at home all day and parents struggled as best they could with very little assistance from anyone. The luckier ones were offered a place at a Junior Training Centre, which was a type of occupational day centre run by the Health Authority. On the whole, these centres were based on nursing care and any educational content was quite minimal.

In 1971 the climate began to change a little: children who were once considered ineducable were now thought to need the benefits of an educational service, and the emphasis was shifting from a predominantly medical model to one that went beyond caring and nursing. The idea of 'training' was to be replaced by 'assisted learning'. So in 1971 an Act of Parliament decreed that Junior Training Centres would cease to be the responsibility of the Health Authorities and would be placed under the jurisdiction of the Local Education Authorities.

As far as special education was concerned, various Education Acts in the past had always placed children into various categories, on which the whole system of special education was based. Children who were defined in law as being 'blind', 'deaf', 'educationally subnormal', 'physically handicapped', 'maladjusted' and so on were provided with corresponding special schools which the Education Authorities built and maintained specifically to house and educate them—'schools for the blind', 'schools for the deaf', 'schools for the educationally subnormal'. In 1971, therefore, all that was needed was to hand over the Junior Training Centres to the Education Authorities, change their name to 'schools for the educationally subnormal (severe)' and add the term 'severely subnormal' to the legal list of special categories. Educationalists responded by developing specialist teacher training and began to place heavy emphasis upon research into this field. The Hester Adrian Research Centre at Manchester University, under the leadership of Peter Mittler, became a leading light for many.

Ten years later the 1981 Education Act was placed on the statute books. By then some people had learnt enough for them to begin to understand the fruitlessness of simply labelling children. The Act made a point of stating, quite clearly, that children should no longer be categorised and labelled; each individual should simply be given the appropriate support and resources required to meet his or her specific needs. Unfortunately, despite the fact that it is now some twelve years since this Act was passed, Education Authorities throughout the United Kingdom continue to maintain schools and units with special categories, such as 'severe learning difficulties' and 'moderate learning difficulties'. Of course, whilst these schools remain intact, brandishing their categories and labels, education officers and psychologists will continue to attach the corresponding labels and categories to children who have additional needs, just as they have always done, in order to keep the schools supplied with pupils.

Despite the Act, the system has not basically changed and the personalised needs of individuals tend to receive mere lip service. In effect, our special educational services seem to have rooted themselves into a rather static and inflexible process, offering people only what the Authority has available, rather than striving to meet the true needs of each child. In short, they have become more resource aware than needs based. The 1981 Education Act made it legally possible for Local Education Authorities to introduce major changes to the way they made special educational provision, a possibility which, alas, most LEAs so far have not taken up. Clearly, the Act states that every child should be educated within an ordinary school, providing that four conditions are met:

1 That the local Education Authority has taken account of parents views.
2 That this is compatible with the child receiving the special educational provision which he or she needs.
3 That this is compatible with the efficient education of the children with whom he or she will be educated.
4 That this is compatible with the efficient use of resources.

I'm sure it will come as no surprise to learn that the fourth proviso is the one most frequently used to prevent children from attending their local mainstream school.

The 1981 Education Act has spelled it out: in principle, all children should be learning together. Labels and categories of disability are of no help and as such should have been abolished a dozen or more years ago. It repeals all the previous education legislation, which has in the past legally referred to those who have learning difficulties as 'idiots', 'imbeciles', 'feeble minded', 'subnormal'. However, even now, in some of our other Acts, they are still referred to as 'defectives'. The 1981 Act has made it clear that no such name tag is particularly helpful. What is far more important and relevant is for us to discover precisely what support each individual should have, in order to meet his or her own particular needs. The Act also gives you as a parent a greater say in what service your son or daughter receives. If you are not satisfied, you now have the power to appeal to a tribunal and, if necessary, directly to the Secretary of State for Education.

The first step in the whole procedure which leads to special educational provision being made for your child is to begin a formal assessment.

What does a formal assessment entail?

Local Education Authorities have a duty under the Act to identify those children whom they believe may have special educational needs. In reality, most of them rely upon referrals being made to them by various doctors, psychologists, teachers, social workers and anyone else who is in close contact with your child and feels that he or she may require additional educational support. You yourself, as a parent, also have every right to notify your Local Education Authority that you think your son or daughter may have additional needs. To do this, you simply write to the Director of Education in your area, telling him why you think an assessment is necessary. If your child is referred by someone other than yourself, it is regarded as improper for them to do so without first discussing it with you. People working within the Health Authority, such as doctors at baby clinics, have a responsibility under the Act to let you (and the Local Education Authority) know if they think your child has or is likely to have special educational needs. If your child is under two years, he or she may be assessed if you wish.

Usually, assessments are set in motion when the Local Education Authority writes to you about its intentions to assess your child and asks how you feel about that. You are given 29 days in which to reply, and legally an assessment cannot proceed until this time is up. It speeds things up, therefore, if you write back as soon as you can. On the whole, unless you feel that your child has no special needs, it is advisable to go along with the assessment process which, after all, is in your child's best interests. In replying, you also have a right to make your own views known about your son's or daughter's needs and what provisions you feel are required. If you feel it is appropriate and your child is capable, he or she may also write to give an opinion. If you are seeking a placement within a mainstream school with support, then it does no harm to be totally up front about it right from the start. Use some of the points in this book to explain why you think your child would benefit from a supported mainstream placement rather than a special school. Some Local Education Authorities send you a form to complete. If you find this helpful that's fine, but you do not have to fill it in; you may if you prefer simply compose and send your own letter. You may also, if you wish, privately engage any other professional you like and ask him or her to write a letter or report in support of what you want for your child, which you can attach to your own contribution.

Local Education Authorities at this stage ask for written reports on your child from professionals such as a medical practitioner, an educational psychologist and the head teacher of your child's school, if your child is of school age. If your child already has visits from a health visitor, social worker, speech therapist or physiotherapist, then a report is likely to be sought from them, too. As a parent, you have every right to be informed by any one of these people that they intend to examine, observe or test your child and you also have the right to be present if you wish. Be sure to make this clear when you reply to the Local Education Authority's initial letter, and raise hell if it doesn't happen.

Having seen your child, the various professionals have to submit their written reports to an officer in the Local Education Authority. Collecting these reports is time-consuming and some professionals are quite lax in getting down to the job and completing it—it is not unusual for this to take a year or even eighteen months or more. If this happens you must complain to the Education Office and get them to chase the individuals concerned. In many cases, parents have quite justifiably insisted that the whole procedure be started again if it has taken too long, since there is likely to be a significant difference between your child's needs and abilities eighteen months ago and what they are now. Under the 1981 Education Act, the Secretary of State for Education has made it clear that a statement of your child's special educational needs has to be completed within a six-month period.

Once these reports have been received, assuming that your child is considered to have special educational needs, the Local Education Authority must produce a document which is called a statement. As parents, you are entitled to receive a copy of each of the full reports that have been written about your child. Usually the Local Education Authority will send you these copies along with a statement or draft statement.

What is a statement and how does it work?

Statementing is the formal process by which a legal statement is made defining what your Local Authority considers to be your child's exact special educational needs and what provision it intends to make in order to meet them. The whole idea of having your child 'statemented' was designed by the 1981 Education Act to be of benefit to children. Unfortunately, in practice it is often used by Local Authority officers to dispense the cheapest and most convenient service, rather than the most effective way of meeting your child's needs.

So how should these statements work and how do they work? Well, a statement is a document which is made up of five main sections. Section 2 and Section 3 together constitute a legally binding contract, so you need to be totally satisfied about what is written there.

SECTION 1

This is simply basic general information, such as your child's name and address, date of birth and so on.

SECTION 2

You will need to look at this more carefully. Remember, this and Section 3 are enforceable by law, since they form the basis of a legal contract. Section 2 is where all your child's special educational needs should be identified and stated. Far too many statements issued by Local Education Authorities are very vague when it comes to this section. This is often a deliberate ploy since the Authority has to write in the next section precisely what provision it intends to make properly to meet the needs that have been outlined in this section. It follows that if the Authority is vague enough about what your child needs, it can also be vague about the intended provisions. So be careful and do make certain that your child's special needs are all fully accounted for in Section 2. Phrases like 'This child requires provision suitable for a child with severe learning difficulties' are completely useless and should be challenged. Section 2 should state clearly and precisely what your child's special educational needs are. References to a 'general developmental delay' or the fact that the child has Down's Syndrome tells you nothing about his or her real needs. It is important that you refrain from giving your consent to a statement which contains key phrases that are woolly, generalised and/or vague. Make certain that, in this section, what is written relates to your child's needs and not to provision. If in Section 2 you find sentences like 'This child needs a special school', then oppose it. A special school is a provision not a need. You need to ask why the Authority thinks your child requires a special school in order to discover what it thinks his or her real needs are.

SECTION 3

Should state specifically what resources the Local Authority will make available to ensure that your child's special educational needs (as described in Section 2) are properly met. Again you must be on the watch for statements that are too vague or general. Sentences which include words such as 'regular' are not acceptable. You may be pleased to find that your child is being provided with 'regular additional support', but you need to know precisely what the support consists of and exactly what 'regular' means. Does it mean every hour, every day, once a week or once a year? What the Authority writes in this space is not a simple promise that can be broken due to insufficient funding. No, what is entered in Section 3 *must* be provided by law.

SECTION 4

Entered into this section is the name of the school (or other arrangements) which the Local Education Authority thinks is appropriate for your son or daughter. You must be certain in your own mind that the school that is nominated will in fact be the most advantageous placement for your son or daughter. Ask yourself: Is the school in the same locality as where you live? Will your child be able to make friends with other children there who are not disabled? Look at the needs of your child as they have been stated in Section 2. If, for instance, one of your child's needs is to develop speech and the school mentioned in Section 4 is a special school, then you will ask how your child can possibly learn how to speak when none of the others in the class or school can talk. When will your child ever hear or participate in normal chatting?

SECTION 5

This deals with any additional provision that your child might need, which is not of an educational nature—for example, speech therapy, physiotherapy, occupational therapy and so on. This whole section is a very loose one. Local Education Authorities have no duty in law to make the provision that is written here. Since provision of this kind is largely under the jurisdiction of the Health Authorities, most Education Departments shy away from acknowledging any real responsibility. The legislation does, however, enable Education Authorities to make this provision if they wish. Not many choose to take up the offer. The sad fact is that you cannot even force the Health Authorities to cover this provision if they choose not to. Nevertheless, it is worth negotiating for, and any Health Authority worth its salt will try to make a reasonable attempt to give your child some access to the various forms of therapy which he or she may need; but don't be surprised if it doesn't add up to very much.

* * *

Once you have received your statement or draft statement, having read it through extremely carefully you will be expected to let the Education Office know whether or not you are satisfied with it. If you are not, then write back saying so, as soon as you can. You do not have to say why at this stage, merely that you do not find the statement acceptable and would like to talk to someone in authority. Once you have done this, you will be contacted by an officer from the Education Department who will invite you to meet him to discuss your objections. If you do not respond within a couple of weeks the Authority will assume that you are in agreement, so you need to act quickly. When you receive your invitation, make sure that:

1 You are clear in your own mind about what you disagree with and why.
2 You are clear in your own mind what it is that you want for your child.
3 You arrange to have someone whom you know and trust to go with you and take notes.
4 You try to predict what arguments are likely to be made against your case so that you can think up the counter-arguments in your favour.
5 You read Chapter Seven of this book.

If after this meeting your differences are not resolved to your satisfaction, ask for another meeting to include those who have contributed reports with which you disagree. Make certain that you take someone along to this meeting who can assist you in making your case—an educational psychologist from outside the area, perhaps, or an experienced head teacher who is not employed by this Authority and who will help you stand your ground. Organisations like IPSEA, Network 81 or CSIE (addresses at the end of this book) may be able to help you in this respect.

At the end of the day, your Local Education Authority may still decide to issue the statement as it stands, but this does not have to be the end of the story. Many parents go on to appeal to the Independent Appeals Panel and are successful. To do this, you simply write to the Director of Education saying that you wish to appeal formally against the statement of special educational needs proposed for your child and give your reasons why. You will have to give more detailed reasons at the appeal itself and so you are advised to be suitably supported and well rehearsed.

You will be contacted to arrange a mutually convenient date and the appeal itself will probably be heard by about five people who will include councillors from the Education Committee or their representatives and someone with a knowledge of special education. In short, this committee is hardly likely to be independent in the real sense of the word, but at least its members will not have been involved in your child's assessment, nor will they be officers from within the Education Department that produced your child's statement. They may well find in your favour, so give it your best shot. The hearing itself is kept relatively informal. You will have a good opportunity to present your case. If you think the whole thing is likely to be far too nerve-racking for you, take a large swig of tonic wine and get someone else to put your case. It is a good idea to take a short video (no more than five or ten minutes) of your child, simply to focus the attention of the appeals committee (without actually saying so) on the fact that it is your child who is under discussion, not a mere statistic. If you can't run to a video, then a photograph will achieve much the same effect. You will probably not know the outcome on the same day, but are more likely to get a letter or phone call telling you of the result. Should this not be what you were seeking, then, if you have the stamina, you may if you wish appeal directly to the Secretary of State for Education. This has proved to be quite successful for some people. The Secretary of State has the power to overturn decisions made by your Local Education Authority and to give you what you want for your child.

Annual reviews

Once your child's statement is in place, it cannot be amended by the Authority without some consultation with you. The Local Education Authority is obliged by law to review your child's circumstances and progress every year. The head teacher of your child's school is responsible for seeing that this happens and any self-respecting school will invite you to be present, along with an officer from the Education Department and anyone else closely connected with your son or daughter. You should be given copies of any written reports (in advance of the meeting, preferably) and you may if you wish write your own comments that you may want to share. By the end of the meeting the head teacher should pull together the views of those present and produce a summary which will be sent on to the Education Office with a copy to you. This review summary will be attached to your child's statement as an update. Where appropriate, there is no reason why your son or daughter should not also be in attendance at this annual review.

The object of the annual review is to ensure that the provision allocated to your child still meets his or her needs and to set new aims and goals for the following twelve months. If you, or an officer of the Authority, thinks that significant changes to your child's special educational needs have taken place, then a reassessment can be set under way. This means going through the whole procedure that you went through to get your child's first statement completed, so as before it is likely to take several months at least. The outcome may be an amendment to your child's original statement, such as a change of school, for example. Annual reviews can in fact be called at any time by you or an officer of the Authority, so don't think that you have to wait a full twelve months before you can make your feelings known. This review is the place where you will have the chance to discuss your child's needs and progress in detail.

When your child is between the ages of 13.5 and 14.5 years, the Education Authority has a mandatory duty to complete a full assessment of his or her needs, unless an assessment has been made within the previous twelve months. The purpose of this is to decide what future provision should be made during your child's final years in school and his or her transition to further education and/or employment. You have the same rights with regard to this assessment as you had with earlier ones.

Keeping a clear vision of what your child really needs

It is quite amazing how negative words like *never* seem to embed themselves readily into the conversation once your child has been described as having a learning disability. Professional people are those who seem to use it, often coupling it with the word *afraid*—'I'm *afraid* your child will *never* be able to . . .' No matter how disabled your son or daughter may seem, he or she will in fact have more in common with other children than differences from them, with basic needs that are exactly the same as anyone else's. Your child will need to know love, have some real friends, reassurance, security and normality in life.

Gloria has a daughter called Ruth whom the experts say has Retts syndrome and is profoundly physically and mentally disabled. Gloria says that she is much like any other child, but she needs additional support that will enable her to participate in all those things which others are able to do automatically. When she was much younger, Ruth attended a nursery school where those who toddled and those who could not toddle played and learned together. Ruth shared the ups and downs of everyday life with her young friends. She had the same choices and opportunities as all the rest. To them, Ruth was simply another member of the class. She got no real extra attention, nor was she ignored or isolated. If Ruth needed something, then there was always someone nearby who could help her. There was always help on hand to move her around, so that she could get from A to B. There was never a fuss made about it: Ruth was simply included in everything that went on.

Then, when they all reached the age of five years, everything changed. Whilst her friends were preparing to go to 'big' school, Ruth's obvious disability caused the system to intervene and send her somewhere completely different, somewhere which they called 'special'. The other children were excited about going to their new school; some were a little apprehensive, but at least they would all be going together. But not Ruth. She was made to travel a different path, in quite a different direction, without the others. Whilst most parents readily recognised that infant school would be a big step for their children and that they would need some reassurance and a little preparation for the adjustments they would have to make, Gloria had a hard time trying to explain to those in authority that Ruth would be feeling much the same. The fact that she had profound disabilities did not mean that she would feel any less anxious when one day her friends were no longer around and she found herself in completely different surroundings, with completely different people. The only real difference was that Ruth could not so easily show her anxiety. Any odd movements or strange sounds that she made were always put down to her disability.

The system ushered both Ruth and her mother onto what seemed to them to be a roller-coaster of events. They soon began to feel they had very little control over all the things that were happening. Chats with psychologists, doctors and education officers left Gloria feeling that Ruth somehow had to be 'fixed', made better, improved upon. It was obvious to her that Ruth's disabilities were going to be a permanent feature of her life, but being unable to walk or talk should not in itself prevent her from going through life with friends and interests or from being a part of things.

They were asked to visit a special school and were assured that it would be exactly what Ruth needed. Gloria arrived there with her daughter, feeling quite nervous and unsure about what they would find. It was in fact much like any other school, except that they had some difficulty getting through the car park where a number of buses were trying to turn and get out without colliding with one another. The buses were there to deliver the children to school. Getting through to the front door was pretty chaotic, but they managed to make it safely to the entrance, where they were met by a pleasant, middle-aged woman who asked them to take a seat outside the head's office. To add to the confusion outside, a team of Council gardeners arrived in a wagon and began to unload a large mower for cutting the grass. Staff passed by, shuffling groups of disabled children from minibuses into their respective classrooms.

Gloria and Ruth had not seen so many disabled children together at one time and the spectacle was quite awesome for them. Gloria could not help focusing on a much older disabled girl who was making a great deal of noise and arching her back in an attempt to free herself from the constraints of the straps in her wheelchair. A staff member caught sight of Gloria watching and explained that they had to ignore her when she did this, because it would otherwise reward her bad behaviour. Gloria smiled back at the member of staff without actually saying anything in response. Inside, she was wondering if this was a glimpse of things to come for Ruth.

The head's door opened and Gloria and Ruth were invited in. A cup of coffee was offered and accepted and the secretary disappeared to make it, leaving them alone to talk. They had only got into the first few sentences when the telephone rang and, realising that the secretary was away making coffee, the head reached over to answer it, apologising to Gloria for the interruption. It turned out to be a member of staff calling to let the school know that she was unwell and not able to come to work for a day or two. Putting the phone back on the hook, the head explained, with a faint note of exasperation, that this was the fourth such call they had received today, which took her total staffing from eight teachers down to six and from six classroom assistants down to four. Again she apologised to Gloria for the interruption and opened her door, calling across the hall to a teacher. Gloria listened as she heard the head quickly explain the sickness situation and suggest that a couple of classes should double up until replacements could be found.

After some discussion, during which all the school's special facilities were brought to Gloria's attention and various details about Ruth were taken down, Ruth and her mother were shown to the classroom where she would be allocated a place, if in fact she came to the school. Gloria was introduced to the class teacher, a small woman with glasses, who smiled at her welcomingly, bending down to say hello to Ruth and doing her best to hide her frustration at having to cope with two classes that morning. 'It's not always like this,' she explained rather apologetically. Looking round, Gloria could see that it was what they call a 'Special Care Unit'. All the children were profoundly disabled and most of them were being lifted from their wheelchairs in order to be placed upon huge bean bags set out in a circle. They were being made ready for the music group that always started the day.

Gloria saw that the older child whom she had watched while waiting outside the head's office was in this class, and after one or two questions she discovered that the group Ruth would be joining had an age range of five to eleven years. Special schools don't have sufficient numbers of children to provide age equivalent classes, she was told; instead they have 'family grouping'. However, none of the other children in this 'family group' could walk or talk. There was no constant chatter of little voices or pattering of tiny feet and none of the busy play that Ruth had been used to in her mainstream nursery school.

Gloria watched as tambourines and other percussion instruments were placed in each child's clenched hand. Ruth was offered one. The teacher began strumming on her guitar and the two other adults burst into song with 'The Wheels on the Bus Go Round and Round'. They moved about between the children who were completely mute, motionless and sinking fast into their deeply filled polystyrene seating. Staff walked between them, stopping every so often to take hold of their arms and waggle them in time to the music. In order to get some response from the children, the staff were singing loudly directly into their faces and striking their instruments close by their ears. One youngster seemed to grimace and contort his whole body across his bean bag, and Gloria was told that this song was his favourite. Over on the other side of the room, the older disabled girl was beginning to shout again and the staff reminded each other that she had to be ignored.

As soon as Gloria had left the special school, she telephoned the head of her local infant school and asked for an appointment. After a lot of explaining and a lot more pleading, she managed to persuade the head to give her daughter a place in the school for just one day each week, to see how things went. To begin with, she had to promise to be there with Ruth. What a difference! For one day a week at least, Ruth found herself back in the thick of things, being pushed in her chair from one place to another, kissed, stroked, and given 'wheelies' in the playground. The children continually stopped to talk *to* her, not just *over* her like many less understanding adults. Unlike the professionals, the children simply regarded Ruth as a person, not as a problem.

As time went by Ruth attended her local school more and more and her special school less and less. There were lots of battles to be fought, of course, and from time to time Gloria became quite exhausted with it all. However, it was plain to her that most of the stress in her life was caused less by her daughter's disability than, ironically, by the type of special services that had been proposed and designed to help her.

Gloria and her daughter had quickly learnt what we all need to learn—that INCLUSION means 'with', not just 'in', and that inclusive education is for everyone. No matter how disabled they may seem, people become more disabled when they are not included.

Don't let your own child become ready, willing and disabled. The system of separate special schooling prepares children for a disabled life which need not exist. It prevents them from experiencing everyday events and routines that other children experience. It takes them away from their own neighbourhoods and local community. It makes it difficult for them to acquire friends, isolates both the children and their families. It stigmatises them, reinforces other people's prejudices and leads them to nowhere in their personal future. They become condemned to lead a life apart from everyone else.

No matter who they are and no matter what degree of disability they may have:

All children need to share normal experiences with other children their own age.

All children need to have neighbourhood friends and relationships.

All children need to have their own identity.

All children need to be valued.

All children need good models of learning.

All children need to learn how to care for each other.

All children need to have equal opportunity.

Inclusive education is not just a way of building better futures for those children who have additional needs, it is about building better futures for us all. When we have an education system that teaches us to recognise the giftedness in each other and how to collaborate to overcome our problems, that's when we shall all have a better quality of life.

If you are struggling with the powers that be to find a place for your child in mainstream education, don't give up, no matter how despondent you may become. Get the solidarity of others around you, form a parents' group and support each other in your efforts. At times it will seem as though you are hitting your head against a brick wall, but remember: if enough people hit their heads against a brick wall it will eventually fall down.

5 Ever-increasing Circles of Friends

'The worst solitude is to be destitute of sincere friendship.' Francis Bacon

When Lorraine failed to turn up for school one morning, the other nine-year-olds in her class were immediately aware that she was missing. Lorraine's considerable physical and intellectual disabilities meant that she could not easily get into her classroom without a lot of help from her friends. So between them the other pupils made a point of ensuring that one or two of them would always be around the entrance just before school started, to greet Lorraine and manoeuvre her through the playground to her place in class. So on this particular morning Lorraine was conspicuous by her absence. The word soon got around and there were murmurs of genuine disappointment.

A few years back, before she had left her special school in order to attend the one at the top of the road like her brothers, Lorraine's mother had harboured fears that her daughter would become the butt of pranks and jokes, perhaps be bullied or simply ignored by children in an ordinary school. That had been three years ago; now Lorraine's mother had no such worries. In fact from day one Lorraine had received more offers than she needed to help her in all sorts of ways—to get her coat on and off at playtime, to feed her at lunchtime and help her with her individual programmes of work—in fact she was included fully in everything that happened.

Whilst all the children helped Lorraine in some way, there were three or four in particular who became much closer friends. These children spent time with Lorraine after school hours and in the holidays. They visited Lorraine's house and she visited theirs. It was these youngsters who taught Lorraine's parents that their daughter was truly a person in her own right and, as such, needed space away from mum and dad at times so that she could begin to embark upon a lifestyle of her own. In the early days it was her young friends who continually challenged Lorraine's mother and father. They didn't realise they were doing it at the time, of course, but Lorraine's parents were themselves very aware of it.

In the past, Lorraine had always attended a special school, where transport had been provided from door to door. When she arrived home she sat in her wheelchair with a number of favourite things on the tray in front of her, and waited for tea to be cooked. Her brothers were usually out playing somewhere. Suddenly, after Lorraine started at her local school, children were calling in and asking if she could come back to their house for tea. Lorraine's mother would answer,

'I don't think so, not tonight.'

'Why not?' the children would ask, and Lorraine's mother would babble something that they all knew didn't make very much sense. The other children's simple invitation had in fact quite floored her. The truth was that she had grown used to looking after her daughter by herself. No matter how tired she felt at times, she had always coped and couldn't really bring herself to trust anyone else to 'see to' Lorraine.

'Perhaps some other time,' she smiled, but quite innocently the children persisted.

'She won't be late back, honest!'

'I think your mother will be too busy to have her round tonight.'

'We've already asked and she says it's all right as long as you agree.' Lorraine's mother searched for other reasons.

'I have to feed her very carefully because she can't chew easily and she might choke if it isn't done properly.'

'We know all that, Mrs Smith. We feed her at school every day and help her onto the toilet and watch out for her fits and . . .'

Lorraine's mother began to run out of reasons why it shouldn't happen and was forced to fall back on her last resort.

'Well, I'll have to phone your mother and see what she says, but I don't think she will be able to have Lorraine tonight.'

When these everyday casual invitations started to happen, Lorraine's mother felt that she had to make a point of phoning and explaining that her daughter was *very disabled* and did they realise that? Invariably she found, to her surprise, that they would say something like:

'Oh yes, we know all about Lorraine. My daughter has been talking of no one else. Don't worry, we'll give her some tea and get her back by 7 p.m. You don't mind her coming here, do you?'

Over time, the realisation came that Lorraine was now simply doing what any other child of her age did as a matter of course. Lorraine's parents loved her dearly, but they had somehow not imagined that anybody else would want her for a friend. Now they were beginning to see what an awful way of thinking that had been. Why shouldn't other people like to spend time with their daughter? On the first few occasions when Lorraine was playing out, her mother was taut with anxiety. It was all she could do to stop herself phoning when Lorraine was just a few minutes late. It was only when all had gone well on several occasions that Lorraine's parents could accept that there was no reason why their daughter should not have her own circle of friends, just like anyone else. Looking back, they can see how they had, without realising it, become one of the major barriers to their daughter living an everyday life.

So, three years on from when she had first begun to attend

her mainstream school, Lorraine's failure to arrive was noted straight away. Her classmates blurted it out to their teacher as soon as she came in.

'Miss, Lorraine's not here.'

'Oh yes,' she replied, 'I meant to tell you. Lorraine's mother phoned to say that she will be in hospital this morning to be seen by the specialist, who may decide that Lorraine should have an operation on her legs.'

Questions from the children came fast and furiously. They talked to their teacher and they talked amongst themselves. Then, as a sort of deputation, they went to see their teacher at playtime and asked,

'Is Lorraine having an operation because it will help her to walk, or is she having an operation to make her legs look like our legs? If it's simply to make her legs look like ours, then we want to say that we're happy with them just the way they are!'

In just three years, Lorraine had not only made friends, she had also gained a strong group of advocates of some thirty children, who wanted to make it clear that their friend should not suffer an operation merely for cosmetic reasons. They like her just the way she is.

The circle exercise

For all of us, life is largely about relationships. The ramifications, consequences and knock-on effect of our daily intercourse with a whole range of people is the very stuff which moulds our behaviour, characteristics and personality. The wide success of TV soaps like *Coronation Street* indicates that what interests us all is the making, the breaking and the cementing of relationships. Take the opportunity of relating to people away from us and it would be difficult to imagine what life would be like.

Whilst most of us can take the notion of socialising and friendships pretty much for granted, many people who have a learning disability find that they have severe limitations imposed upon them, by their families and by a whole range of professionals, through the separate services that are provided by them.

Marsha Forest and Jack Pearpoint have introduced an interesting exercise which they call the circle exercise. Apply this process to people who are your son's or daughter's age and you might well find it most enlightening. It may also help you to gain a better insight into your own son's or daughter's current circumstances. Start by asking them to draw a series of four circles all inside one another, just like Figure 6. Then ask them to write down their name in the centre and, on the line of the innermost circle, ask them to write the names of those who are closest to them, the people whom they love and who love them (as in Figure 7). Then proceed to the line of the second innermost circle and have them write the names of those people whom they like a lot, friends of whom they are fond but who are not as close to them as those they have placed in their innermost circle. Then, on the line of the third circle, ask them to write the names of contacts and acquaintances they come across in their life through being a member of the same club, organisation or church—people whom they meet fairly regularly every week or every month (see Figure 8). Finally, on the line of circle number four, the outside circle, ask them to write down all those people who are paid to be in their life, like teachers, doctors, hairdressers and so on (as in Figure 9).

Whilst they are going through this process, do the same with your son or daughter so that you are able to compare the circle patterns of both at the end. For many people who have learning disabilities and are enforced by various special services to do things separately from the rest of us, once you take away those people who make up their family, those who are paid to be with them and those who also have a disability, there are often none left. Figure 10a shows a typical circle which has been completed by a person who is disabled and using special services. Figure 10b, in contrast,

Figure 6

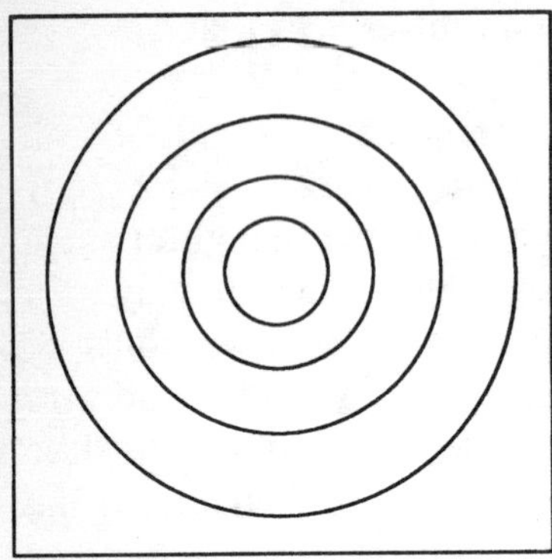

Figure 7

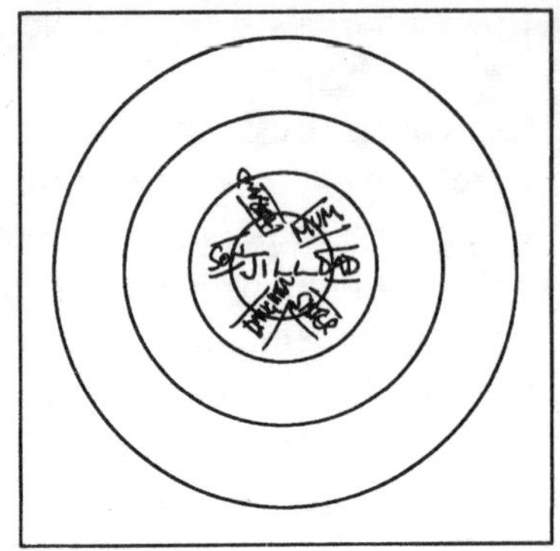

Figure 8

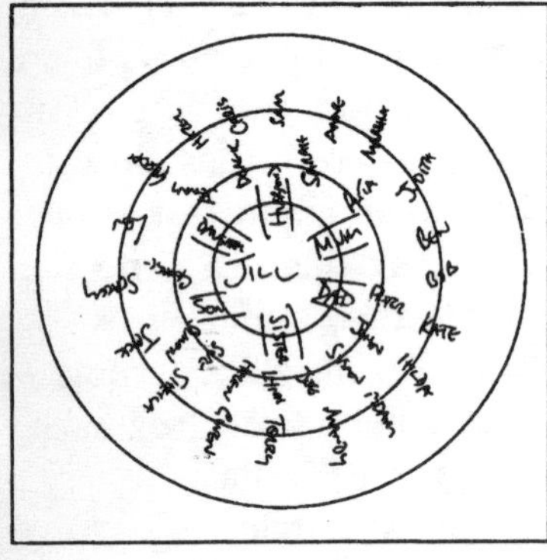

Figure 9

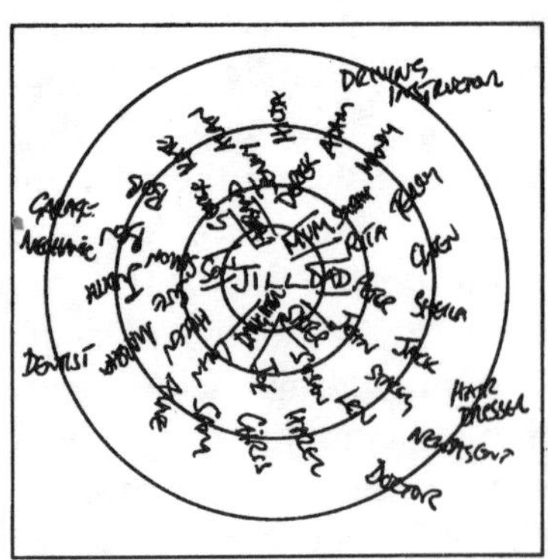

Figure 10a

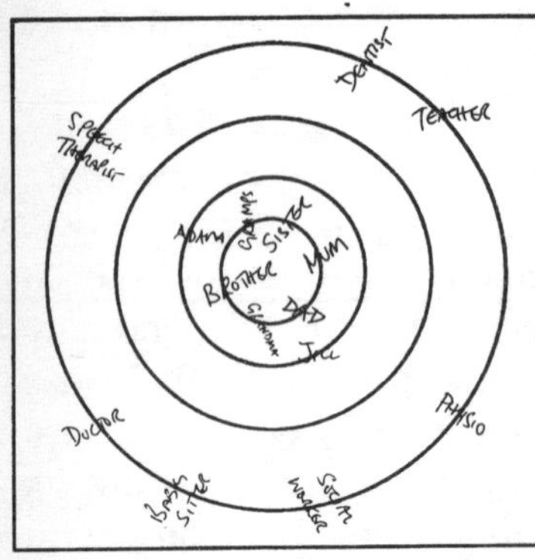

Figure 10b

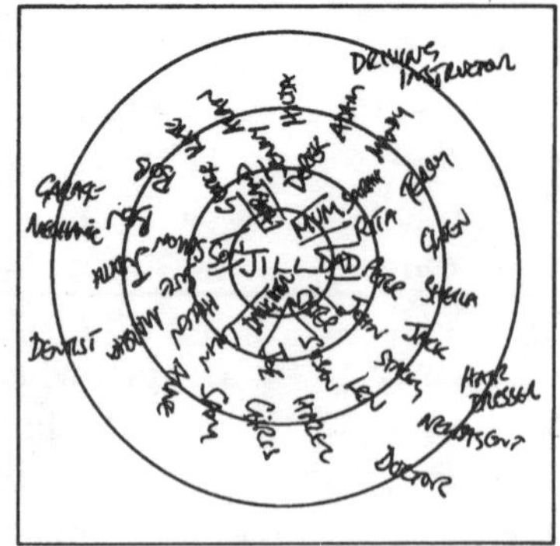

Figures 6–10b. *The circle exercise.*

shows a typical circle completed by someone who is non-disabled. Too often, people who have learning disabilities have circles which are either barren or sparse in their second and third circles, as in Figure 10a.

If you stop for a moment and ask yourself what your life would be like and how you would feel if your circles looked like that, you will begin to have some idea of the poor quality of social life and companionship that many disabled people are largely stuck with. Marsha Forest took a group of twelve-year-olds through this exercise and at the end of it asked them that same question. Their answers were quite typical:

'I'd commit suicide.'
'I'd act mean.'
'I'd do bad things.'
'I'd be scared to death.'
'I'd act stupid.'
'I'd die.'

Creating a circle of friends

We learn about friendships right from our early years. School becomes a great catalyst for us, where we get wide opportunities to meet others of our own age who live in the same area as ourselves. Each of us learns how to make judgements about others, whether we are attracted to them or not, whether we get on with them easily and how we resolve any conflicts that we may have. We discover that if we are to make any friends at all, we have to start to consider what they like and may want to do as well as contemplating our own preferences. School is an experience which enables us to choose people to whom we best relate and to experiment with various interests we can share. So, in relationship terms, what happens for most of us quite naturally and informally may need, initially at least, to be created somewhat artificially for those people who have learning difficulties. If, because of their disability, they have been placed in a special facility which prevents them from having much contact with their non-disabled peers, they will not have had the same chances in their formative years to build these kind of relationships.

A CIRCLE FOR YOURSELF

Creating a circle of friends for your son or daughter may actually start by creating a formal circle of friends for yourself. No one stands alone for long in this world. We all need support to make our accomplishments and if you want to help your son or daughter live a full life, you in turn will need help to make this possible. For some reason, most of the time we try to struggle on with tasks which are quite obviously beyond our ability to cope with alone, and yet we rarely consider asking others for help. We do so only as a last resort. If our car breaks down in the high street and won't move an inch forwards or backwards, we tend to push our hand through the driver's window in a futile attempt to steer the vehicle with one hand and apply our shoulder at the same time to move the brute. Whilst we would never dream of asking for help, inside we are praying that someone in the traffic hold-up that we have caused will stop hooting and cursing and come over to lend a hand. Perhaps it is a British trait, but somehow we always seem to feel that we have to go it alone. Often we are too concerned that asking someone to get involved may cause them too much awkwardness if they want to say no. So we never ask, and in this way we prevent others from joining us. Whilst we don't like to ask for help, in the same way, others who would love to give their assistance feel that we may not want them to offer. In opening the door of opportunity for your son or daughter, you will probably need a small group of people around you, who can give you that added strength and confidence.

THE INVITATION

Starting such a circle couldn't be simpler: you only have to ask. A group of five or six people is a good manageable number and they can be almost anybody. They can be friends already, or members of the family, or just acquaintances. They can even be people whom you do not know. If you have difficulty in thinking of half-a-dozen people, then simply ask two and get each of them to bring with them two other people they know. All you are asking of them is to come to your home one evening for coffee and to spend an hour or two helping you to think of a few answers to some problems you have in making your disabled son's or daughter's life fuller and more interesting. Make it clear that you are not asking them to get personally involved in a hands-on way, but merely to brainstorm some ideas and form part of a small group who are going to think as creatively as they can. You are asking them to commit just a couple of hours for this. People are more likely to give up their time if they understand that there is a limit to what is being asked of them. It is worth making it clear, too, that they are not expected to have any sort of qualifications, but simply to help you think through some ideas.

THE FIRST MEETING

It is useful to have a large sheet of paper on the wall, on which you can write or draw symbols that represent the group's thoughts and the suggestions people make. The bigger the sheet of paper the better. If you do not have enough wall space, then the floor or a table will do, so long as it is the focal point of the group and everyone can see it easily. Your first task is simply to thank people for coming and say that you would welcome their help in thinking out some ideas that you hope will benefit your son or daughter. Introduce your child either by having him or her present, which is the best option, or by showing a five-minute video or half-a-dozen photographs. Then ask everyone in the room to introduce themselves if they are not known to each other. While they are doing this, write the heading 'Who's Here?' and draw a simple figure with the person's name attached (see Figure 11). You don't have to be Leonardo Da Vinci, the simplest drawing will do. As time goes on, you will see

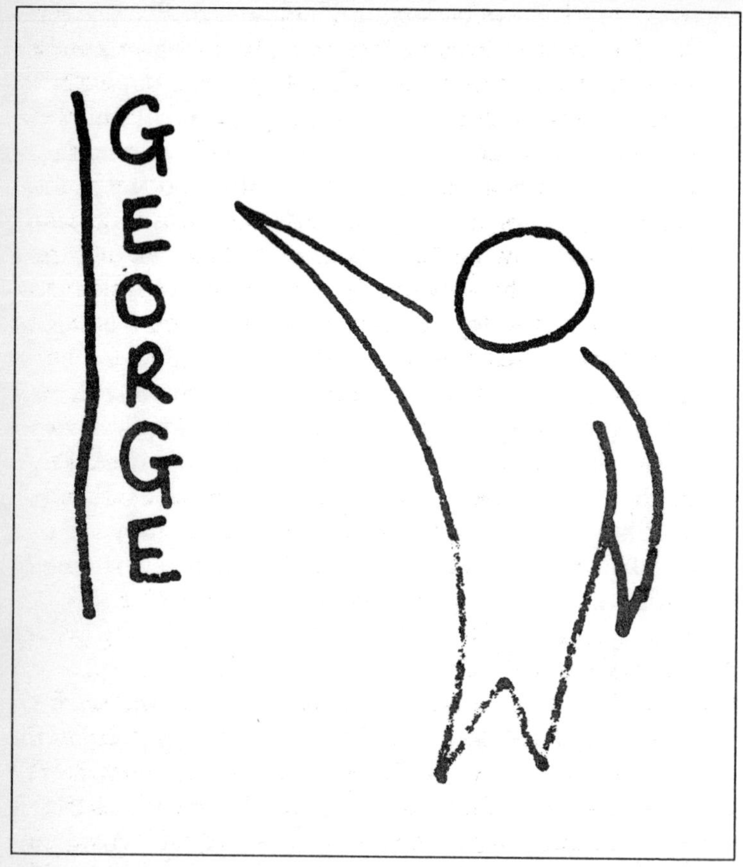

Figure 11.

that the rest of the group respond well to this way of recording. Write down the key word or phrase that they use, it gives them a feeling that what they say is valued and will encourage them to have more dialogue.

Then comes the real start. Say something about your child, what sort of person he is and what has happened in his life so far. Have your partner or someone else continue with the graphic recording as you speak, drawing or writing the salient points. A typical introduction might go as follows:

Our son John was born nine years ago and during that time has always lived in this area. He is a lively little boy who loves music, drawing and playing with other children. Like a lot of children his age he sometimes gets overexcited and he can be quite naughty, too. Most of the time he is a cheerful lad who enjoys being in the centre of things and always tries his best to please people. Just now his biggest craze is dinosaurs and he spends a lot of his time poring over books and pictures about dinosaurs, trying to trace them and playing with small models that he is collecting. Life has been quite difficult for him at times because he is not yet able to speak very well and the fact that he has Down's syndrome has meant that the Local Education Authority has provided a special school for him to attend some eight miles away. Of course, because all the other children in his school are also disabled, John's speech is not helped because he doesn't hear much in the way of normal talking. This leads to him getting quite frustrated and upset sometimes. Although he has lived here all his life, because he has to go to school outside the area John hasn't had a chance to make any friends of his own age locally. He is home by half-past four most school days and then doesn't have any friends to play with. The same applies to every weekend, and of course he is on holiday for three months of the year. We would like to see him become more involved with children around here so that he can have a fuller life and have more friends. We're not sure of the best way to do this because John doesn't seem to have much of a chance to meet the children around here and they don't know him. We were hoping that by getting a few people together tonight we might be able to think of ways in which we can make this happen for him. It doesn't seem a lot for a nine-year-old lad to ask . . .

Then ask the circle to throw in any ideas they can think of which might help. It doesn't matter how incredible or impossible they sound; start by getting as many ways of overcoming John's problem as you can. You can sort them out and hang on to the best ideas as you progress.

By encouraging others to help you in this way, you will find that the circle starts to take on a momentum of its own. People begin to get excited and enthusiastic once they begin to see the possibilities. Remember, you are not asking anyone actually to do anything other than think up ways of creating opportunities to improve your child's life. Of course, you wouldn't stop them if they did want to make a bigger contribution. Try to be specific: it will help others to focus their creativity. For example, you may ask them to think of ways in which your son or daughter could find five friends by this time next month. Using a group to generate problem-solving ideas and to use their own contacts and acquaintances is always more effective than continually trying to do it alone.

STARTING A CIRCLE OF FRIENDS FOR YOUR SON OR DAUGHTER

It doesn't matter whether your youngster is of school age or an adult, he or she will still need to have real friends of her own. If she hasn't yet managed to develop a full circle for herself, then helping her to get under way is one of the most useful things you can do. Your circle of support will give you plenty of ideas about where your child can go to meet others of her own age. It is in one or more of these places that your son or daughter may need to have a circle established. If she is of school age, her own classmates are a good place to start. Once again you will need to make the simple invitation. Perhaps it is better made via the class teacher, once he or she understands what is required.

'We are looking to create a circle of friends for Jane so that she can get the opportunity to do all those things that everyone else in this class does—go to the cinema, join the guides or youth club and so on. We are looking for about eight or ten of you to join Jane's circle of friends and meet together with her and me once a week, to discuss what is needed and plan how we can make it happen.'

I have not yet met a class who didn't respond well and enthusiastically to this simple invitation. Over time, of course, various members of the circle leave and new ones come into it. This is the same for us all. Think how boring it would be if we all maintained only the same friends that we started with throughout our whole life. In a more formalised circle like this you can always have the understanding that should someone wish to discontinue, he or she has the responsibility to find a replacement. The idea of the circle is that each member will not only discuss and plan together, but will also each play an active role in accompanying Jane to and from places where they already go and introducing her to their friends. This way Jane has the opportunity of expanding her networks of friends and acquaintances in a variety of places. Any potential difficulties in doing this, and the logistics involved, are to be discussed and tackled by Jane's circle of friends. Any difficulties you may have in coming to terms with this can be sorted out and chewed over with your own circle of support.

MAPs

One framework to use in getting some group cohesion and encouraging members to focus clearly on the issues is a facilitation exercise designed by Jack Pearpoint, Marsha Forest and Judith Snow. They refer to it as MAPs. Once again, you will need to begin by putting a lot of paper on the wall and drawing out the diagram shown in Figure 12.

1 WHO'S HERE?

Even if everyone knows each other quite well, still begin by getting them to introduce themselves and perhaps say a line or two about why they are there or what they feel about it. As each person speaks (your son or daughter will of course

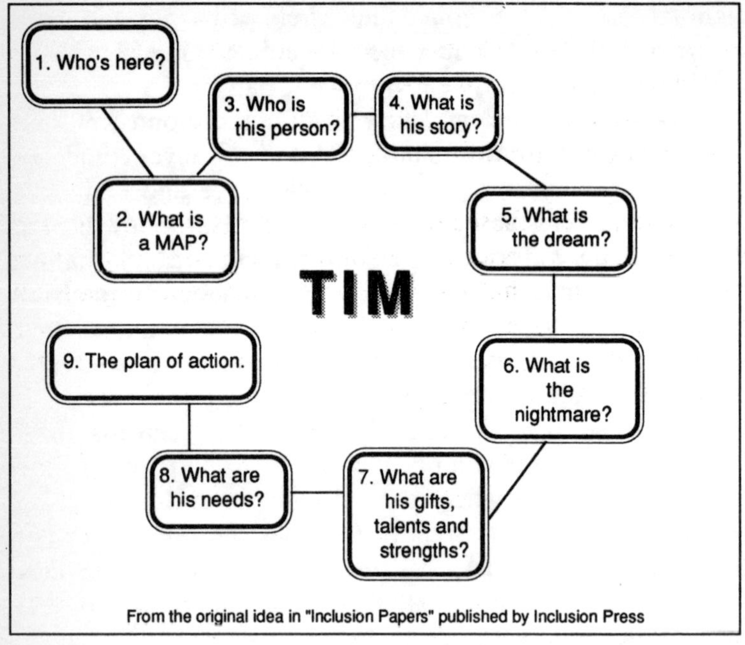

Figure 12. *The Layout of a MAP* (Pearpoint, Forest and Snow)

also be present), make a simple illustration in number one box on the diagram to represent what he or she says, or write down the odd word or phrase that records his or her contribution. Be sure to include everyone and try to use what they say verbatim. This way people will be encouraged to contribute and feel that what they have said is valued. Of course, circles of friends can include just about anybody who wants to be involved and groups are often made up of a mixture of children and adults together.

2 WHAT IS A MAP?

Once the introductions have been made, you or whoever is facilitating the group should move on to circle number two and ask, 'What is a map?' Again, write down the answers that people call out. They are likely to be things like:

'It gets you from A to B.'
'It helps you to plan a route.'
'It shows you where the barriers are.'
'It shows you what direction to take.'

You can then use these answers to point out that the process that the group is about to use is called a MAP for the same reason—namely, that you are going to attempt to get from A to B, plan a route, try to anticipate the barriers and decide what direction to take in making Tim's life (for example) more full and interesting for him.

3 WHO IS TIM?

Following the same procedure, ask the group to give you a thumbnail sketch of Tim's character. What sort of person is he? I can tell you that those in circles that I have facilitated have never yet described the person concerned as disabled or handicapped. They always express things like:

'He's cheeky.'
'He sulks sometimes.'
'He enjoys being with other people.'
'He has a good sense of humour,' and so on.

In special school situations and other similar segregated services, when I have asked staff about a particular person in the same way, very often they seem to accentuate negative factors and concentrate more upon the things the child is not able to do well.

4 WHAT IS TIM'S STORY?

Then ask, 'Where was Tim born?' and 'How did he come to be here?' This is usually where parents or other family members give most of the answers and in doing so often considerably enlighten the others who make up the group. They will not have experienced or even thought about the difficulties that you will have encountered in bringing up your child. Most people assume that parents who have a disabled child are given considerable help and support by various Local Authority services. Listening to how you were told about your child's disability may well be an eye-opener in itself. How long was it before you were told? How sensitively was it done? What real practical help were you given afterwards and since? During this session, people in the group may well learn things like:

'Once a week I had to take Tim to the specialist. This meant an hour's journey from our house to the hospital taking Tim and his two brothers, who were both under five years, on three buses to get there. Then we would usually have to wait around for about an hour before seeing the doctor who spent about ten minutes asking us how things were going.' Or:

'We were so frightened when we brought Tim back from the hospital. We weren't sure how we were going to cope with his fits. Neither of us slept very much for months.' Or:

'Until he was five, Tim had always played with the other children who lived nearby. He went to playgroup with most of them. Then, when it was time for them all to go to big school, Tim was sent several miles away to a special school whilst all his friends went to the school at the top of the road like his brothers.'

Only a few weeks ago, when I was facilitating a MAPs meeting, in order to try to gain a place for a child in her local mainstream school, I could see the amazement and sympathy being expressed on the face of the head teacher of the local school who had been invited to be a member of the group. On hearing the child's history, he became extremely motivated and determined to offer as much help as he could. Reading school and medical reports in their clinical form is one thing; listening to the human story told by parents, brother and sisters can be quite another.

5 WHAT IS THE DREAM?
Now, in circle five, continue to record the group's dream for Tim. What is it that they want for him? They are likely to offer answers like:

'For him to have lots of friends.'
'For him to be happy.'
'For Tim to go on to the secondary school with them.'
'For Tim eventually to live in his own house with companion helpers.'
'For Tim to get a job.'

This section helps the group to become bonded and build together a shared vision of the future. It encourages them to take ownership of the responsibility for helping to make Tim's life as rich and full as they can.

6 WHAT IS THE NIGHTMARE?
Similarly, by recording their worst fears of how Tim's life could turn out, means that the group can begin to foresee some of the pitfalls to avoid, so that they can ensure that the nightmare never happens. Each group is different, of course, and will generate different thoughts, but will often answer with phrases like:

'That he has to live in an institution.'
'That he has no friends and becomes very isolated.'
'That he never gets invited anywhere.'

7 WHAT ARE TIM'S GIFTS, TALENTS AND STRENGTHS?
In this section record all the things that, in the view of the group, Tim has going for him and refer back to them when it comes to making the plan of action in circle number nine. In one group, for example, they were trying to think what job their friend could do when he left school. This was not easy since he was completely paralysed, unable to speak and had considerable intellectual difficulties. They tried hard to

come up with the things that he did well. Amongst other things, they decided that what he did really well was to sit still. After all, he was paralysed, so sitting still was one of the few things that came quite easily to him. They racked their brains to see how this could be useful to an employer and finally came up with the idea of helping him to apply for a post as an artist's model. He now earns a living doing just that.

8 WHAT ARE TIM'S NEEDS?

Again, working collaboratively, Tim's friends will be reinforcing their commitment as a group and recognising all the factors that cause gaps in his life compared with other people's, if they are not fully attended to.

9 THE PLAN OF ACTION

Of course each plan of action will be different, but it will be arrived at by consensus of the group and through a process of collaboration. As they meet each week, the group will need to refer to their MAP, so it is a good idea to keep it somewhere prominent. It is not, however, something to be treated as if it were carved on stone and can be changed whenever the circle of friends feels it necessary. Reviewing the MAP is a useful thing to do, and from time to time, particularly when members of the circle come and go, a fresh MAP will need doing.

* * *

Whenever I have been asked what I would wish for if I was granted just one wish, I have always replied that I would wish that I had another three wishes. I asked the same question of a young woman with Down's syndrome whom I met in the West Country recently. She thought hard for a moment and then said, 'To keep my friend.' My curiosity got the better of me and I asked about her friend. It seemed that she had known someone called Helen since they were children. Now that they were both in their mid-twenties, having left school they no longer saw each other every day. Because they lived about eight miles from each other, it wasn't easy for them to get to one another. Although now a young woman, she was not allowed by her parents, with whom she still lived, to travel on the bus by herself, and in fact someone whom she called her key worker did his best to prevent her from meeting up with Helen. It seemed that Helen was known to lose her temper quite easily and would throw things. They were concerned that she might get hurt.

I asked her if Helen had ever thrown anything at her. Most emphatically she answered 'No'. When I asked if Helen had ever hurt her in any way, she again said 'No'. Then she went on to explain that she had always been able to calm Helen down in her times of stress and that she had always been the one who could talk to Helen and explain that she was only getting herself into trouble by losing her temper. She would hug Helen and soon her anger and frustration would subside. They had been each other's friend for several years. Now, for her own good, she was told, they were being kept apart. She didn't know what was happening to Helen these days and was concerned for her. She had no other friends in her life, only her immediate family and her key worker. So when I had asked her to make one wish, it was not for wealth or health or happiness, but simply to keep her friend Helen.

The problem that disability often brings is that it can insist that you have to rely so much on other people to enable you to do the simplest task. For some people disability means always having to stay in one place until someone else decides if and when it's all right to take you to another place. For some people disability means being unable to tell others what they want and how they feel. It means being pushed from here to there, never knowing when or where you are going; being left at a place and never being told when someone will come back for you. Disability for some means being treated as a child throughout your whole life. Being disabled can mean rarely if ever being listened to. This is why true friends are so necessary.

A circle of friends may have to be engineered somewhat artificially in the early stages, but with care it will grow into an ever-expanding network of people who don't merely do things for your son or daughter, like voluntary workers or paid personnel, but who develop the elements of real friendship, whereby both parties gain from a reciprocal arrangement; whereby they do things together, sharing an interest; whereby they rely upon each other, learn to trust one another and achieve give and take on both sides.

Too many people will want to measure your son's or daughter's progress by how well he learns to walk or talk, read or write, when what will matter most is that he has a quality of life enriched by a circle of true friendships, one which enable him to be a part of his community, to live the life he loves and to love the life he lives.

6 Your PATH to a Better Future

> 'Jumping at several small opportunities may get us there more quickly than waiting for one big one to come along.' Hugh Allen

Keeping a clear sense of purpose and direction is something which most of us find difficult to accomplish, particularly in relation to our own day-to-day existence. We all need to have some idea of what we want out of life and what we want to put into it. We have to have some idea about what will make us happy, in order to find out how we can go about achieving it. The trouble is that most of our efforts seem to be taken up just dealing with all the everyday mundane tasks which we continually have to address in order to survive. Time ticks steadily on and often, before we realise it, we have shuffled into yet another decade, without doing any of those things we once dreamed so much about.

Marsha Forest and Jack Pearpoint, along with John O'Brien, have been developing a process which can help people to focus on their hopes and dreams and then to think out practical ways in which they can make those dreams come true. The process is called PATH which stands for Planning Alternative Tomorrows with Hope. The process can be used in all sorts of ways. It can become a planning tool for organisations to give themselves a clearer picture of what they want to achieve and how they might go about achieving it. It can be useful to couples, to enable them to communicate their thoughts, ideas and wishes to each other about how to get the best out of their lives and relationship. It can be used by businesses large or small, by voluntary organisations, families or individuals.

Used in conjunction with the MAP framework (described

in the previous chapter), the PATH procedure can be a practical tool for making positive future changes. As in the MAP process, ideally two independent facilitars are required, one to introduce the process and to guide it, the other to record graphically what each person is contributing. There is no reason why these two roles should not interchange throughout, and indeed any members of the group should be made to feel that they can involve themselves at any time with the graphic recording if they wish.

The PATH process

A PATH starts by inviting people to come together, who share a common cause or interest or who want to solve a common problem. Sometimes people don't know that they share a common problem until they actually do come together. You may also invite people to share common hopes and dreams. In the next section of this chapter, 'A PATH for Nikki', it was Nikki's parents and younger sister who brought together a class of children, teachers and a head teacher to plan with Nikki the shape that his life might take in the following year.

PATH is a social process and maximum diversity within a group usually achieves better results. Nikki's PATH consisted of people of all ages and backgrounds, professional and non-professional, men and women, family and friends. The members of your group cannot see things from a different perspective if everyone is a teacher or an adult and has the same view from the start. Therefore, the number of people who become involved in a PATH is quite immaterial. I have facilitated a PATH involving just two people and I have also facilitated for groups of forty-plus. However, most PATHs seem to be conducted with around six to ten people participating. As in MAPs, the facilitators will need to have a supply of coloured felt-tipped pens, a sheet of paper about 6′ × 4′ and of course a wall or floor space large enough to display it for everyone in the group to see. On this paper the facilitator will draw the shape of a large arrow pointing into a circle, as shown in Figure 13. Do not include the words 'Step 1', etc.; the graphic recorder's task is to fill up these areas of blank space with words, phrases, symbols and drawings which are meaningful to the group and which make an accurate record of what people contribute and communicate. The PATH process

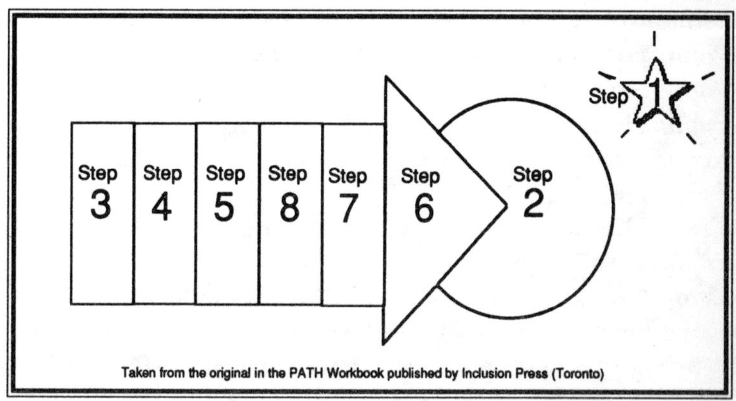

Figure 13.

involves taking people through eight clearly defined steps:

Step one: The North Star
Step two: Making goals
Step three: Where are we now?
Step four: Who do we need to enrol?
Step five: Making ourselves stronger
Step six: Targets for the next few months
Step seven: Next month's work
Step eight: Taking the first step

A PATH for Nikki

To help me to describe these steps in more detail, those involved in Nikki's PATH, which we did recently at his school, agreed that I could use their experiences to illustrate the process in this book. To begin with, I used part of the MAP sequence to get people to say who they were and why they were there. I then explained that I had never met Nikki before and that he had never met me, so I knew almost nothing about him.

Kenn: I want you to tell me more about Nikki by using just one word to describe him.
Pupil: He's jolly.
Pupil: He's exciting.
Pupil: He's a bit noisy.
Kenn: How else can we describe Nikki?
Pupil: He's giggly.
Kenn: Oh, he gets the giggles sometimes, does he?
Pupil: He's happy.
Kenn: Good, give me some more words that describe Nikki. We have already said that he's jolly, exciting, a bit noisy, he's giggly and he's happy, and . . . what? *(Pointing to a group of adults.)* Somebody over here give me a word.
Adult: I am curious.
Kenn: That describes you, now describe Nikki.
Adult: He's intriguing.
Kenn: Does anyone know what intriguing means? *(No answers.)* Well, if someone or something intrigues you, it means that you want to find out more about them. Just one more word that describes Nikki.
Nikki's dad: He's cheeky.
Kenn: So is this a fair description? We've said that Nikki is jolly, he's exciting, that he's a bit noisy, he's giggly sometimes, he's happy, intriguing and cheeky. Is that fair enough? Does that tell us what you think Nikki is like? *(General nods of approval.)* I want to find out now how Nikki came to be where he is today. So I'm going to ask members of Nikki's family about this. *(Looks over towards the family.)* Can you tell us something about what you experienced when Nikki was born? How did you find out that he had additional needs?

Nikki's mum: When he was born, Nikki had real feeding difficulties. Nikki didn't swallow like other babies did.

Nikki's dad: He didn't sleep very well either and he would take an hour or two to feed.

Kenn: So how did Nikki come to be in this school?

Nikki's mum: We just approached the headmaster.

Kenn: What concerns did people have about Nikki in those days?

Nikki's dad: That he couldn't speak and that he couldn't eat very quickly. The other alternative was for Nikki to go to a special school.

Kenn: Has anybody here ever been inside a special school?

Pupil: Yes, I have.

Kenn: What was it like?

Pupil: The corridors smelt like a hospital. My brother used to go to one.

Kenn: What is a special school?

Pupil: A place where you go when you are disabled.

Kenn: Why doesn't Nikki go to a special school? *(No answers.)* Well, why does Nikki come to this school?

Pupil: Because he will learn just as much here as he would at a special school.

Kenn: Right, let's move on now.

STEP ONE: THE NORTH STAR

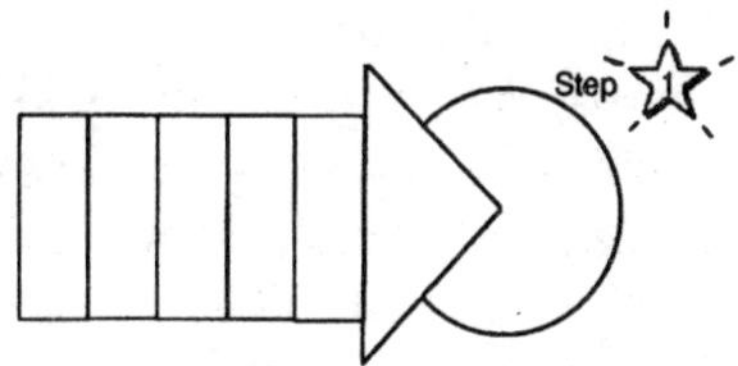

At this point I moved into step one of PATH, which was to get the group to decide what they wanted for Nikki in the very long term. This is where the group defines the North Star for which they are ultimately aiming.

Kenn: When you eventually leave school and become grown-ups, what things will you want for yourselves?
Pupil: A decent life.
Kenn: Good. And what is a decent life? What does that mean?
Pupil: To have a good future.
Kenn: Right, and what is going to happen in your good future?
Pupil: To be able to help people.
Pupil: To have lots of money.
Pupil: To have a family.
Pupil: To have a happy life and not a sad life.
Pupil: To have a good job.
Kenn: What would be a good job?
Pupil: One where you don't have to work too many hours. *(Laughter.)*
Kenn: Like a teacher, you mean? *(More laughter.)* What else do you want when you're grown-up?
Pupil: To be successful in my job.
Kenn: Right. That's great. So, when it comes to Nikki, what is your dream for him when he grows up?
Pupil: I'd like him to become like a normal person.
Kenn: Tell me what that means.
Pupil: I mean that I want to see him get a normal job like everyone else. A proper job where he earns good money.
Kenn: Good. What else?
Pupil: I want to see him lose all his disabilities.
Kenn: Which ones does Nikki have at the moment that you want to see him lose?
Pupil: So that he can talk better.
Kenn: OK. What else?
Pupil: I want to see him lose his learning disability.
Kenn: Anything else?
Pupil: I want him to be happy.
Kenn: That's good.
Pupil: I want him to get married and have a family.
Kenn: Where would you like to see Nikki living?

Pupil: In a normal house with normal people. The same sort of house that Nikki is living in now.

Kenn: Perhaps we can get his mum and dad to sell it to him cheaply. *(Laughter.)* What about Nikki's mum and dad? What is your dream for Nikki in the long term future?

Nikki's dad: All those things that the children have said; brilliant.

Kenn: Do you have anything else to add?

Nikki's mum: I'd like to see him get more choice in his life.

Kenn: More choice—right, good, what else?

Pupil: That Nikki has friends and is not ignored by other people or on his own all through his life.

Kenn: Yes, I would hate that, wouldn't you?

Pupil: To have a proper house. I don't want him to be on the streets.

Kenn: So, what you are saying, then, is that your dream for Nikki in the future is to see him lose some of his disabilities, perhaps talk better and get more independent as time goes on, so that he can look after his own life more and have more choice. You would like to see him get a job and live in a normal house. You want him to have friends and not be alone or ignored. Is that OK? *(General nods of approval.)*

STEP TWO: MAKING GOALS

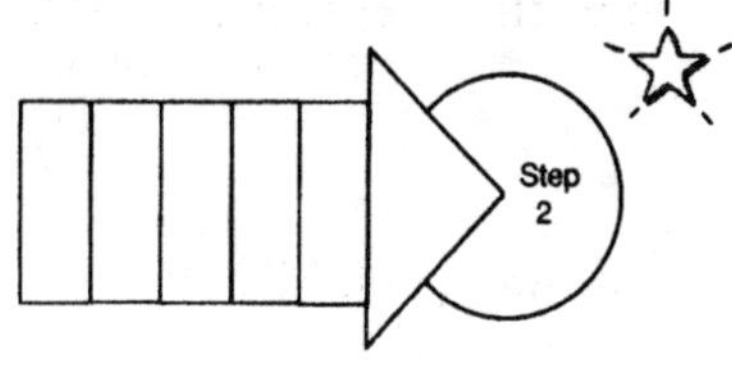

This is where the facilitator gets the group to share their dreams for the next twelve months in particular. They have to be specific in what they would like to see happen within the next year. The facilitator has to make certain that the group propose targets which are both positive and possible to accomplish.

Kenn: What we are going to do this afternoon is a thing called PATH. This is a PATH *(points to the paper on the wall where the group's answers so far have been graphically recorded)*. PATH stands for Planning Alternative Tomorrows with Hope. If Nikki's life is always to get better and head towards these long-term hopes, wishes and dreams that you have for him, then you need to decide what should be happening for him in the next twelve months. So I want you now to imagine that this classroom which we are sitting in has turned into a time machine, like the one Dr Who uses. We can now travel so fast that we can go forwards in time. Close your eyes and hold on to each other tightly because we are about to travel very fast indeed. When you hear me clap my hands, open your eyes, because you will then have landed and it will no longer be the 7th September 1993 but 7th September 1994. *(A hand-clapping sound is made and the group open their eyes.)* OK, we've arrived. Do you remember me coming here and speaking to you a year ago? *(The group grin and nod their heads.)*

Pupil: Yes, we shared our dreams for Nikki.

Kenn: Well, a whole year has gone by now and I heard that you had a very good year indeed. In fact I heard that everything has gone really well and it's been brilliant. Tell me about some of the very good things that have happened with Nikki.

Pupil: Nikki still lives at home.

Pupil: Nikki has lost some of his disabilities.

Kenn: Which ones has he lost?

Pupil: His talking.

Kenn: So Nikki is able to talk better now, is he?

Pupil: Yes.

Kenn: How is Nikki speaking better?

Pupil: He can say more words.
Kenn: How many more words?
Pupil: Fifteen.
Kenn: Good. What else has happened in this really good year?
Pupil: He doesn't need as much help. He can walk on his own.
Kenn: So how is Nikki able to walk better than before?
Pupil: He can go places on his own now, when he used to have to go with somebody else before.
Kenn: Good. Which places? Tell me one or two places that Nikki is now able to go, that he couldn't before.
Pupil: Over to the fields from the classroom.
Kenn: So Nikki can now go over to the fields without help from anyone else?
Pupil: Yes.
Kenn: What else can Nikki do now?
Pupil: He has more choices.
Kenn: What sort of choices has Nikki now got?
Pupil: He's started to choose his own clothes.
Pupil: He chooses what he eats.
Nikki's mum: Nikki can feed himself at home now. *(She laughs and explains that she is told that Nikki feeds himself at school but she still has to do it at home.)*
Nikki's dad: Nikki is toilet trained.
Kenn: So Nikki can now tell you that he needs the toilet and has far fewer accidents?
Nikki's dad: Right.
Kenn: Any more good things happened? *(No replies.)* Right, so Nikki in this great year that has just passed can now say fifteen more words. He can walk over to the fields without any help. He has become toilet trained and he can feed himself at home as well as at school. On top of all that, Nikki has more choices in his life and is choosing what clothes he wears and what he has to eat. So it really has been a very good year indeed. *(Everyone smiles.)* Now that Nikki can do all these things that he couldn't do last

year, how does that make everyone feel? Give me one word.

Pupil: Glad.

Pupil: Happy.

Pupil: Cheerful.

Pupil: Fantastic.

Adult: Great.

Kenn: Give me one more word, somebody.

Adult: Ecstatic.

STEP THREE: WHERE ARE WE NOW?

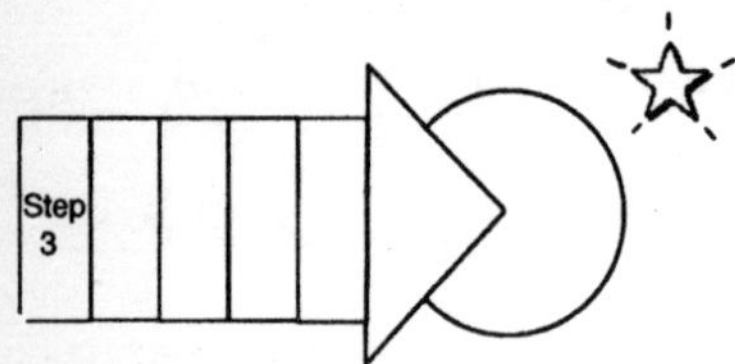

At this point the facilitator needs to make the group realise just where they are now in relation to making their dreams for Nikki come true. They have to see what life is like for Nikki in their own terms and allow this to motivate them to tackle things together on his behalf, so that he can have a chance of becoming the Nikki that they were dreaming of just a few minutes ago. This step allows them to see what is possible for Nikki and to understand that these possibilities are in their hands: what the future holds for Nikki will depend largely on them.

Kenn: OK, let's get back into our time machine, hold tight to one another and close your eyes because we are now going back through time until we all arrive safely back here, today, 7th September 1993. Here we are, and none of your dreams for Nikki have happened yet. Nikki doesn't choose his own clothes or food. He needs other people to help him to walk. He can't say very many words.

He doesn't feed himself at home and he is not yet toilet trained. So how does that make you feel at this moment?

Pupil: A bit sad.

Pupil: Helpless.

Pupil: Nikki is not as happy as he should be.

Kenn: Any more?

Adult: Dependent.

Kenn: So you have a way of measuring how successful you are in achieving your dreams for Nikki not by testing him or assessing him but just by knowing how you feel. If you are feeling a bit sad, or helpless, or if you feel that Nikki isn't as happy as he could be, then you know that you haven't got very far, but if you feel glad, happy, cheerful, fantastic and great, then you know that you are getting somewhere.

Pupil: It doesn't have to be a dream, does it? We could make it happen.

Kenn: Right, so everything that you've just dreamed about and would like to see happen for Nikki in the next twelve months is perfectly possible, if you as a group try to do something about it. Let's look at how it could be done.

STEP FOUR: WHO DO WE NEED TO ENROL?

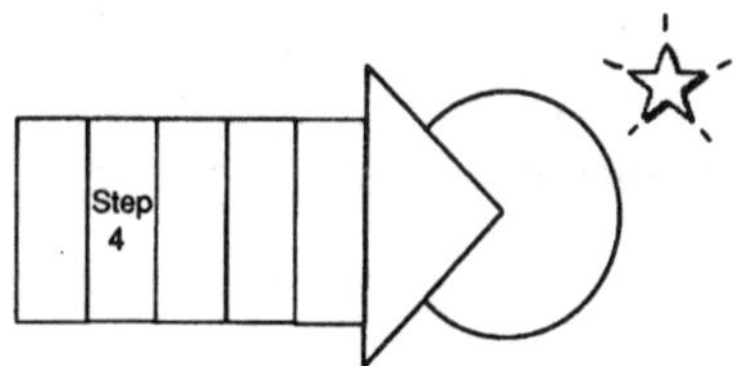

Now the facilitator should select any one of the goals from step two that have been recorded to achieve a year from now, and begin to get the group to put some practical flesh on the bones by encouraging them to consider what help they can get to make this particular goal happen.

Kenn: Let's look at what you want to happen for Nikki by this time next year. You have said that you would like him to:

1 Choose what he eats.
2 Choose what he wears.
3 Be able to walk to the fields without help.
4 Be able to say fifteen more words.
5 Become toilet trained.
6 Be able to feed himself at home.

Which one of these shall we start with?

Pupil: Number five.

Kenn: So if Nikki is to be able to look after himself properly on the toilet by this time next year, who do you need to call on to help you with that?

Pupil: All of Nikki's friends.

Kenn: OK, anyone else?

Nikki's dad: Mum and dad.

Nikki's sister: His sister.

Pupil: Mrs Hogan and Mrs Williams *(Nikki's specialist helpers in school).*

Kenn: Do we need anybody else? *(No reply.)*

STEP FIVE: MAKING OURSELVES STRONGER

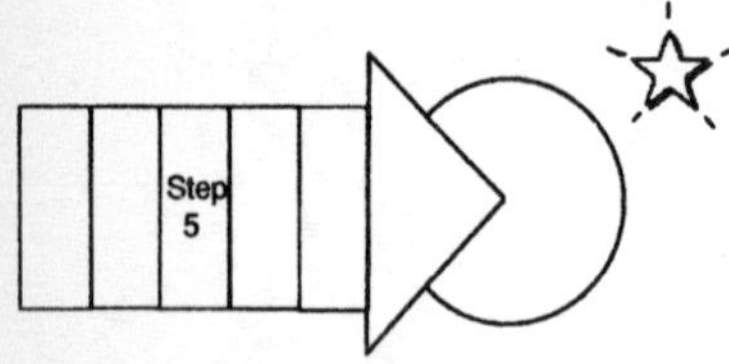

Next the facilitator asks the group what sort of things will make them strong enough to see the task through. So often we fail to accomplish something simply because we are too tired, or fed up with doing it, or don't get any credit for doing it. This section recognises that it is the simple things in life, like this, that are so important and can make the difference between success and failure. Step five has been built into the PATH process so that these things can be recognised and accounted for.

Kenn: We all need different forms of support to enable us to see a job through. Sometimes we need to make more time, or sometimes we just want to hear encouragement from our friends to continue. What sort of things will make you feel stronger and more able to cope?

Adult: I think we need to keep reminding ourselves about the goals that we want to accomplish for Nikki so that we don't let it just drift into doing less and less.

Kenn: That's a good idea.

Adult: We need to keep a chart of some sort to show how well things are going.

Pupil: We could take five minutes at the end of class on a Friday afternoon to talk about how it's all going.

Kenn: That sounds fine, any more? *(No replies.)*

STEP SIX: TARGETS FOR THE NEXT FEW MONTHS
and
STEP SEVEN: NEXT MONTH'S WORK

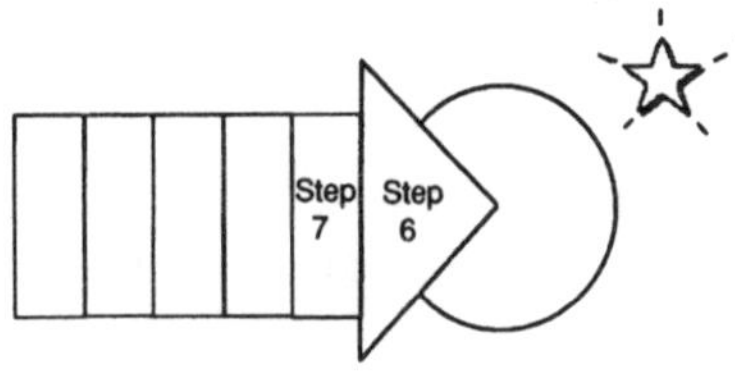

At this stage the facilitator gets the group to break down what they want to have achieved in nine months' time, or six months' time or three months' time, in order to be on target for reaching their goal in a year from now.

Kenn: If Nikki is to become toilet trained by September 1994, then what sort of things should he be able to do by this Christmas?

Adult: By Christmas he should be able to indicate to people that he wants to use the toilet.

Kenn: How will you get Nikki to do that? What will he need to have learned by October?

Adult: Well, Nikki will have to get into a regular routine of being taken to the toilet throughout the day.

Kenn: So how possible is that? Nikki will have to be taken out of class five or six times every day to visit the toilet and get into a routine.

Class teacher: There would be no obstacles to prevent that.

Kenn: Who could do that?

Class teacher: Well, his special member of staff is here and there are the other children in the class.

STEP EIGHT: TAKING THE FIRST STEP

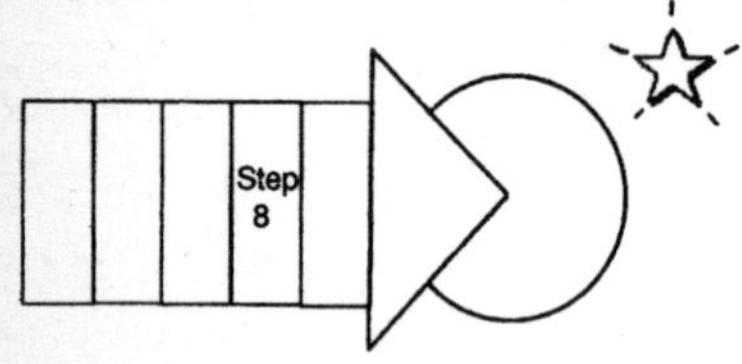

Finally, the group have to consider what their first step will be if they are to reach their goal. Things have to start somewhere or nothing will get done at all.

Kenn: Right, then. If Nikki is to be able to look after himself on the toilet a year from now, by Christmas you want him to be letting others know that he wants to use the toilet. And for Nikki to be doing that, you have said that by next month he will be in a routine of having people take him to the toilet six times each day throughout school time. So to set all that going, what do you need to do to take your very first step?

Pupil: We need to know what times Nikki is going to be taken to the toilet.

Kenn: Good. Who is going to sort that out?

Adult: I'll do that.

Kenn: Fine. What else?

Adult: We need to know who's going to take Nikki at each different time. *(Several children put their hands up to volunteer.)*

The PATH is completed when the group have been taken through each of the other five goals that they have made for Nikki. This need not always be done at one sitting but could be completed in a number of sessions if necessary. Nikki's PATH was concluded as follows:

Kenn: How many people think that the dreams you have talked about today are important for Nikki? *(Everybody puts their hands up.)* So if they are important, what will you have to do more of to see that they actually happen?

Pupil: Include him more.

Pupil: Help him more.

Pupil: Welcome him.

Pupil: Encourage him.

Kenn: How much is all that going to cost you?

Pupil: Nothing.

Kenn: Nothing at all. So you can all afford to do it. I'm going to leave this PATH that you have made for Nikki on the wall and it will be up to you whether or not it comes true.

Some things a facilitator should bear in mind

a Facilitators are independent and must not come with their own hidden agendas. Their key task is to get the group to bond, and to assist them in finding solutions to their own problems.

b Get a consensus of agreement right from the start about what time you should finish. For most PATHs you should try to allow at least one and a half hours or thereabouts.

c Your role is to empower people, not to create any form of status or power for yourself.

d The facilitator has to provide the initial energy to get things moving. He or she also has to keep the momentum of the group flowing. So give it plenty of pace.

e Ask relevant and open-ended questions like 'What can be done about that?' or 'What do you need to make that happen?'

f Whilst you will constantly be asking the group thought-provoking questions, do not get drawn into providing the answers yourself. Facilitators are not there to solve problems, they are there to mobilise the group's thoughts and answers.

g Facilitators should not try deliberately to shape any of the answers. This is not your PATH, you are only a custodian of it for others.

h When you are new to it, the PATH process is unknown to you and people can easily find uncertain situations like this threatening. It is the facilitator's task to put people at their ease as quickly as possible. So use plenty of humour; after all, a PATH is a fun thing to do. People in the group should also understand that there are no right or wrong answers, just answers for everyone to share with each other.

i In my experience, significant differences of opinion are very rarely expressed during a PATH sequence. However, should a confrontation occur, then avoid giving it much space or time. Simply assist the parties to work out their common ground by having the graphic recorder draw or write something with which they both agree. If this is not possible, then be sure to record a simple word or phrase from each.

j Do your best to see that everyone gets the opportunity to contribute, as some people are dying to say something but are very shy. Similarly, don't let just one or two people dominate the whole thing.

k Make sure that you continually summarise throughout, by reading out to the group those things they have said which have been recorded graphically.

l Before you facilitate for others, try to make sure that you go through the PATH process personally, for yourself. You need to know what it feels like and to discover how useful it can be.

A few graphic ideas for recorders
(Taken from the work of Jack Pearpoint)

You don't have to be good at drawing to be a graphic recorder. Practice makes perfect, so you will have to be like all other graphic recorders and just take the plunge and do it. You will be surprised at how easy you will find it. You don't have to be silent throughout the whole process. A graphic recorder is also the ears, so you should let him know if he has missed something or heard somebody wrongly. Below are a few ideas with which you can practise, but it is much better to develop your own repertoire. Take some felt tips and a pad and practise by doodling about the things people around you say. All you need is a bit of imagination.

The advantages of making a PATH

The PATH process is valuable because it provides a framework in which people are:

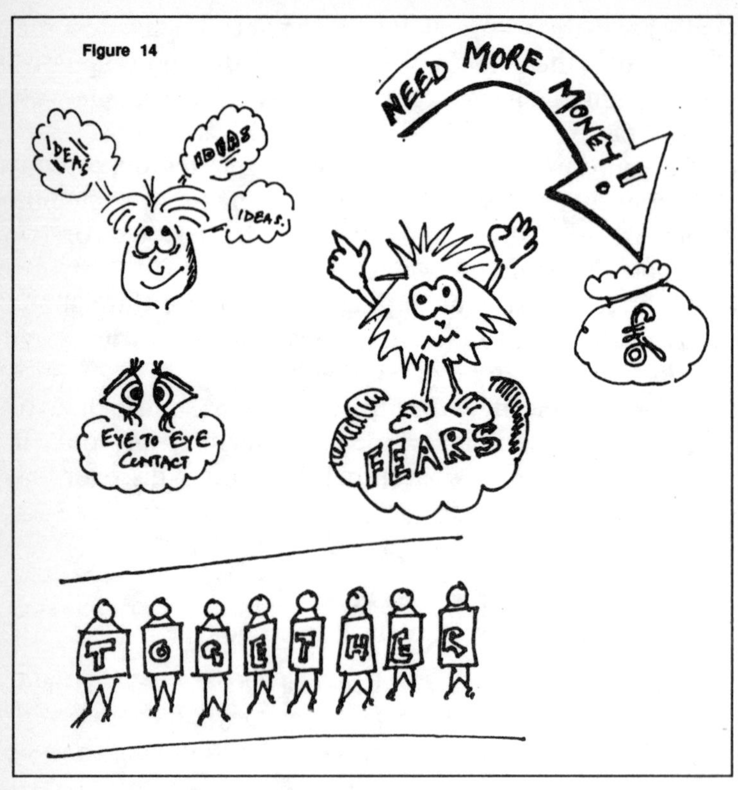

Figure 14

Figure 14.

COMMUNICATING AND RELATING BETTER TO EACH OTHER

Too often people become so polarised in their views that inevitably there is a great deal of friction between them. Eventually, after continual confrontations, a breakdown of communication or credibility occurs. Those who believe strongly in inclusive education, for instance, see themselves as coming up against the brick wall of bureaucracy which always appears to put up barriers that prevent them from realising their goal. As a result they seek to increase all the pressure they can muster against the bureaucrats, to make their wishes happen. In scenarios like this people seem to resort to aggressive vocabulary:

'We will fight the Authority all the way!' or

'We've been battling against the Education Committee for years and we're not giving in now!'

A definite 'us' and 'them' situation is created, with both sides seeing each other as opponents who must be defeated. The effort, energy and resources that are put into long-lasting confrontations of this kind are enormous; they would be much more usefully deployed in efforts to collaborate with one another. Of course, sometimes confrontational situations cannot be avoided, but we do seem to take up these warring positions far too quickly, adopting them as a first option rather than a last resort. Those of us who favour inclusion may see traditional service providers as heartless, budget-orientated bureaucrats who are completely incapable of understanding the real needs of those who have additional needs; the bureaucrats on the other hand see us as evangelical, over-emotional, idealistic extremists, who want to force our views on everyone else and must be prevented from doing so.

The PATH process, however, allows everyone to focus positively on the needs of the person concerned. Right from the start, it shows that everyone's contribution is welcomed and valued and ensures that all parties have the opportunity to communicate their thoughts and ideas in a non-threatening atmosphere which is both collaborative and optimistic.

STEPPING BACK TO LOOK FORWARDS

PATH gives us a chance to take a step back and look at the situation from a different perspective. If we imagine life to be like a millpond, then we know that as people jump in they will create a series of waves, and as more and more jump in, the waves will go crashing in different directions and we become lost in the general turbulence. In order to see our situation more clearly, we need to rise above the millpond and look at our own position from above, where we are free from the turbulence caused by others. In the

PATH procedure, each person in the group can begin to listen to others and see things from a different perspective. The fact is that each of us is a part of the existing problem, and if we are to change things in order to reach a solution, then we ourselves often have to change too. A well facilitated PATH can enable us to see and understand what changes we shall each have to make.

ENGAGING THE EMOTIONS

Many professionals are trained not to get too involved with their clients, and as a result our Human Services often seem to be overseen with an air of detachment. Whether you participate as a friend, a member of the family or as a paid professional, the PATH process will engage a range of your emotions as you listen to the stories and accounts of other people in the group. Once, when I was facilitating a PATH, I saw a head teacher of a mainstream school become more and more shocked as he listened to a mother talk quietly of the time when she was told that her baby had serious disabilities and how she had been waiting for over eighteen months for her son to receive an essential piece of apparatus which had originally been promised within a week. The head teacher had no idea that this could happen; he had always assumed that all the stops were pulled out for disabled children, whom he believed were well provided for and treated as a priority. His sense of injustice led him personally to undertake a whole series of tasks during the PATH meeting, many of which he dealt with the very next day.

Professionals rarely see all that a disabled child and his family experience. Each doctor, psychologist, therapist and so on only ever sees his or her small part of the equation and never really understands what it is like to be on the receiving end of the whole service. Paediatricians, for instance, receive their patients in a clinic at the convenience of their own surgery. Parents are expected to turn up on time, come wind, rain or shine, despite the fact that they may have had to catch two buses to get there, encumbered with three children, all under the age of five. Having overcome this part of the obstacle course, it is not unusual for them to have to spend an hour-and-a-half or more in a waiting-room, trying to keep their children amused until the doctor is ready to see them. The doctor's time is seen as precious and not to be wasted; a mother of three, on the other hand, seems to be regarded as having the lowest status, with the whole day to kill. Similarly, teachers only see the children in their class for a year, at the end of which they are passed on to the next teacher and a new intake is received. They therefore often find it difficult to appreciate what becomes of the children throughout the system as the years go on. The PATH process allows each participant to realise and understand the extent of the difficulties which everyone else has to face, and it does so in a way that is not personally threatening or aggressive.

DIFFUSING POWER

Under normal circumstances, meetings, conferences or reviews are presided over by someone in power. Throughout the proceedings it is recognised that some people wield more power than others. Power is seen as rising upward to the top from where policies, resources, decisions and answers come. The PATH process does not require a chairperson or team leader, but is independently facilitated, which means that power is dispersed and shared by every member of the group, whether he or she is a parent, a nine-year-old child, a head teacher or a director of education. It is recognised and appreciated that each person is valued for his or her contribution and that together much can be accomplished, both simply and effectively.

ESTABLISHING JOINT OWNERSHIP

Going through the experience of PATH together creates a sense of shared ownership between the participants. The personalised group cohesion which becomes established can motivate people to see things through to a satisfactory conclusion and to accept their measure of the responsibility, rather than avoiding becoming directly involved. When it is facilitated well, the process establishes a trust between people and builds a common understanding between them, which becomes a sound foundation from which they can pool their ideas and resources and express their willingness to tackle difficult yet surmountable problems. Each group member's unique contribution is brought together to express a shared dream and form a united response.

7 Speaking up for Them and with Them

> 'No one can make you feel inferior without your consent.'
> Eleanor Roosevelt

On the whole, those of us who make up the public at large seem to be very good at offering charity to those whom we, in the first place, have systematically consigned to a place outside the mainstream of our day-to-day lives. Shaking tins and organising sponsored parachute jumps appears to come far more easily than understanding that what is needed is rights, not hand-outs. Where charity is concerned, there is often considerably more to be gained by those who give than there ever is by those who receive. Charitable giving not only leaves us feeling tingly-warm inside and at peace with ourselves, it also elevates our own status to that of benefactor and philanthropist. Quite frequently it does us no harm to be seen in this light and may be instrumental in our own social and career advancements. So when you get down to brass tacks, those who appear to give in fact receive, and those who appear to receive in fact lose out.

Corporate giving in this way is no different. Some companies that make high-profile gestures of caring may themselves benefit considerably more, in advertising terms or by increased sales of their product, than those who have become the object of their charity.

No doubt you will think this is quite a cynical view to take; what does it matter, anyway, so long as those who are in need benefit? But before you condemn me out of hand, speak to a few disability groups and find out for yourself how they feel when they are portrayed in this way. Ask them if they think that they really do benefit. Whilst events like Children in Need and Comic Relief are undeniably successful in raising millions of pounds, at the same time they take away the dignity of countless individuals by turning them into 'good causes' and 'objects of pity'. Of course, they generate huge income, but they also shape distorted attitudes and perceptions which in the long term are quite counterproductive to the needs of those people whom they purport to assist. Whilst television controllers offer programmes like *Link* and *Read Hear* to encourage disability awareness, other programmes, like *Children in Need*, undermine them in one fell swoop.

It has to be said, too, that charitable programmes of a celebrity nature are allocated hours at peak viewing time, all with able-bodied presenters; conversely, programmes which bring real issues of disability to the fore are relegated to half-an-hour at unpopular viewing times, replacing what the media used to refer to as the 'God Slot'. The message is manifestly clear: our own acts of charity are very much valued and are to be celebrated with fanfares, whilst the rights of people who have additional needs can be quietly acknowledged, providing it does not interfere with the rest of us too much. I have to say at this point that, in television terms, Channel 4 is somewhat the exception. They have understood these pitfalls for some time and have begun to address the situation.

So, in social terms, whilst charitable acts can be an excellent medium through which we can elevate ourselves, all too often these gains are made at the expense of the intended recipients. People who have learning difficulties are undoubtedly marginalised and often depend heavily upon the likes of you and me to lobby, campaign, represent and speak up not just *for* them but *with* them. This means that we have to listen to and understand what *they* want and not persist in doling out what *we* think they need. On the whole, such people are far from influential when it comes to operating within the corridors of power. They generally have a weak voice and are rarely heard. They will almost certainly need our support in safeguarding their interests. To do this, you will need to plan ahead. There will be times for thinking and times for doing and after each action it is always worth sitting back and reflecting upon the outcomes and what you have learned from them before you progress further.

In speaking up for someone, whether it be your son or daughter, brother or sister or a friend, you will need to understand their needs in precise terms. From what you know of them, ask yourself (and them where possible) how life could be better for this person. Make some comparisons between the way that they experience day-to-day living and the lives of many other people of the same age and circumstance, who do not have a disability. Compare their opportunities in things like making friends, sharing a hobby, membership of local clubs and so on. If you find that they are continually segregated from other people in order to spend their time with people who also have a disability, then ask yourself where this is leading. What future does it hold for them? Do people with disabilities really have that much in common just because they share the same label, or are they being prevented from keeping in touch with local people, with whom they could develop a more enabling and satisfying relationship?

Are they having as full a life as other people?
In what ways are they losing out?
Do they have what other people take for granted?
Do they have equal opportunity?
Do they have as much choice as they could?
Do they have as large a repertoire of skills and concepts as they could?
Do all their friends and acquaintances have a disability?
Do others of a similar age who live locally even know that they exist?

How many real friends do they have?

Do they have genuine interests and hobbies which they can pursue?

Do they only belong to clubs which are specially designed for those who are disabled?

Every so often, ask yourself these questions and ask them openly, together with other members of your family and those who are in your circle of friends. You may find it useful actually to write down a clear statement, or perhaps a series of statements, of those things which concern you most about the lifestyle of your disabled friend or relative. If we are not careful, over time we can all adjust our perceptions, attitudes and efforts to fit in with what may in fact become quite a barren life. People who have learning difficulties are at greater risk of gradually having severe limitations placed upon them, quite unwittingly, by those who are closest to them. Often, our notion of disability can take the form of a game of O'Grady. Whilst O'Grady says 'do this and do that', so do we use the concept and the word 'disability' to make ourselves and others do this and do that. Instead of O'Grady says . . . it becomes Disability says . . . and without questioning it too deeply we embark upon a road of unnecessary restriction. It is important to keep making the comparisons of what we would have expected in the same circumstances if our friend or relative had not been allocated the label 'learning difficulties'.

As has been remarked upon earlier in this chapter, sadly, as a society, we seem more comfortable with providing charity than parity for people who have a disability. Inevitably, therefore, there will be times when such vulnerable children and adults will need considerable support in speaking up or will need someone to speak up with them. On occasion, you will find that even the most basic of human rights will have to be fought for. This is not because officers and staff of the various services are inherently wicked; it is more likely to be because they are themselves the product of a segregated education and so have real difficulty in understanding the full picture. Mostly it is these people's distorted perception of disability that causes them to believe that what they are doing is best for their 'clients', 'pupils', 'residents' and 'patients'.

As I travel around the country, meeting and speaking to people in various special services, I invariably discover some really nice individuals who, without realising it, are doing some pretty awful things. The belief of some professionals, that they know better than you, has been instilled into them by their training and by the status afforded to them by others. It is all too easy to be intimidated by the aura of such people, especially when they reinforce their 'authority' by presenting themselves in formal offices and sport the notorious power dress of pin-striped suits or jackets with padded shoulders. It can take a good deal of courage to overcome the barrier of a desk placed between you and the piercing stare of a pair of eyes over the top of spectacles. However, you must have trust in your own judgement and believe in the strength of your own argument in order to achieve the outcome you seek.

Parents and advocates cannot avoid having to deal with professionals, whether they be teachers, head teachers, psychologists, doctors, speech therapists—whoever. The natural assumption we all make at first is that these people are there to help both you and your son or daughter. Well, some do and some don't. Some will and some won't. Some will try to be as helpful as they possibly can and appreciate your situation and anxieties; others, however, will have more concern for their own career prospects and will not want anyone to rock their boat. Such people will see you as an irritation if you do not readily fit into the established system and routines.

The most helpful person is one whom we will call a true civil servant. These people will be both *civil* and will provide you with a *service* to the best of their ability. True civil servants may not always be able to give you exactly what you want, but they will at least try their utmost and have a genuine commitment to being of some service. On the other hand, the bureaucrat will only want to safeguard his own pay cheque and conserve his own best interests.

So how do you tell which is which? Well, there are always a few give-away clues, hidden in the way professionals say things. What they say and what they mean may not necessarily be quite the same. For example:

The bureaucrat will say:

'Well, of course, I realise that your child needs this resource, but I'm afraid there just isn't enough in the budget. There is only one cake, you know, and there are lots of demands made upon it.'

Roughly translated, this means, 'We need all our money for normal children; don't be so greedy.'

The true civil servant will say:

'I understand that your child needs this resource, and whilst we don't have enough money to provide it at the moment, there are at least some things that we can explore together. First we can . . .'

The bureaucrat will say:

'You can't rush these things, it takes time to develop programmes like this, you know.'

What he really means is, 'Don't be so pushy. If you'll just ease up a bit and lay off me, with any luck I can take so long doing nothing that you'll get fed up and forget all about it.'

Civil servants are more likely to say:

'Yes, I'm sorry, I should have done that. I promise you that I'll work on it straight away.'

The bureaucrat will say:

'I'm sorry, but you have to understand that we can't

change the whole place around just to accommodate your son.'

What he is really saying is, 'No chance, we're not changing, we like things the way they are. They have always been like this and we have found it very comfortable for us. You've really got a nerve asking us to change.'

A civil servant's reply will be more like:

'Well, that seems like an idea worth trying. Frankly I'm not really sure that it will work, but if you feel strongly about it we will certainly give it a go and see how it turns out.'

Bureaucrats are those people who:

1 Make you feel that they are to be respected and that you are there to benefit from their expertise.
2 Will try to keep you ignorant of your rights and any facts that will help you but make their job more difficult.
3 Will be personally and professionally offended if you try to make them accountable.
4 Will do their best to avoid involving you fully in planning.
5 Will decline to speak up for you in meetings where other professionals (their colleagues) take a different view.
6 Will blame you or somebody else when things go wrong.
7 Be unable to comment due to 'confidentiality' or 'professional ethics'.
8 Protect themselves first.

True civil servants are those people who:

1 Will provide you with as much information as they can and put you in touch with other individuals and groups who can give you support and advice to enable you to get what you want.
2 Apologise when they are wrong.
3 Recognise your expertise about your child and his or her needs and treat you as an equal partner in planning to meet those needs.
4 Will relate to you as a person and not as a client.

5 Try to build up your skills, knowledge, self-confidence and understanding of all the issues, so that you can be a good advocate for your son or daughter, brother or sister or friend.
6 Welcome the opportunity to answer your questions rather than be threatened and defensive because of them.

Getting organised

To be successful in acting as your friend's or relative's advocate, you will need to be well organised. If you are unhappy about something and want to get it changed, then you will need to know who has the power to make these changes. Who is it that makes the decisions? Who is in a position to make sure that you can get what you want? If you don't make your plea to the appropriate person you are unlikely to accomplish very much. Whilst going directly to the top can be very effective, sometimes it is better first to talk to somebody who knows how the system works, what its infrastructure is and if there is an unofficial network operating which is perhaps more effective than the proper channels.

Making contact

In contacting key people, writing a letter may seem the obvious way of making an appointment, but this is in fact the easiest for them to reject. Telephoning is marginally better, but often it proves difficult to talk directly to the person you want as there may be a barrage of clerks and secretaries to get through first, and at the end of it all your conversation may be cut short by your being asked to write in with your query. Face to face is the most effective method of contact since it is the most difficult to reject. In formal terms, you may simply ask the person who you think can help you for an appointment. On the other hand, it may be better for you to invite him or her to be the speaker at a meeting.

Here you would at least know when and where you would be able to talk to him in person and you could even prepare the ground by getting other people in the audience to ask the speaker relevant questions. There are of course more informal ways of making contact, depending on who the person is and what relationship he or she has with you. Inviting your child's class teacher or head teacher for a meal or a drink can be an excellent way of making your views known. You may decide to arrange a 'chance' encounter or perhaps find out who or what influences a person through someone who knows him or her well.

Avoid angry opening gambits

Whether you are attending a meeting or arranging an informal contact, it is rarely worth going in with all guns blazing. No matter how angry you may feel about the situation, make certain that you check your facts with the person first. Ask general questions first to discover what is happening and why. Try to make some assessments about the person to whom you are talking: is he a true civil servant or is he a bureaucrat? How does he perceive the situation? What are his unspoken assumptions about what others are doing and saying? Remember, you could have got your facts wrong, so it is as well to test the ground before you launch into an attack.

Attacks, anyway, only usually serve to put people on the defensive, which means that they are less likely to keep you fully informed of all that they already know. They will also probably become antagonistic towards you—if not to your face, then when you are no longer there. Whenever they become the butt of other people's frustrated anger, bureaucrats will tend to blame you, the victim, rather than acknowledge any failure within their system. The following lists will give you some idea of how various systems are organised and whom you can approach with your concerns or complaints.

SOME POINTS OF CONTACT IN THE HEALTH SERVICE

First talk to the person immediately concerned or the manager of the service. Then try:

- The Secretary of the Community Health Council (CHC)
- The District General Manager at the District Health Authority
- The Citizen's Advice Bureau
- The Local Councillor for your ward
- The Chairperson of the Health Committee
- Your Member of Parliament
- The Secretaries of State for Health and Social Services
- The Health Services Commissioner—Health Ombudsman
- Your Family Practitioner Committee

(Your local librarian or post office will provide addresses for the above.)

SOME POINTS OF CONTACT IN SOCIAL SERVICES

First talk to the person immediately concerned or the manager of the service. Then try:

- The Director of Social Services
- The Local Councillor for your ward
- The Chairperson of the Social Services Committee
- Your Member of Parliament
- The Secretaries of State for Health and Social Services
- The Local Authority Commissioner—Ombudsman

(Your local librarian or post office will provide addresses for the above.)

SOME POINTS OF CONTACT IN THE EDUCATION SERVICE

First talk to the person immediately concerned or the head teacher. Then try:

- The Chairperson of Governors
- The Local Councillor for your ward
- The Chairperson of the Education Committee
- The Director of Education
- The Assistant Director concerned with special education
- The Educational Psychologist

- The Education Adviser for Special Educational Needs
- Your Member of Parliament
- The Secretary of State for Education
- The Local Authority Commissioner—Ombudsman

(Your local librarian or post office will provide addresses for the above.)

Keep a file

Keeping a file or notebook and writing down simple statements about matters that concern you most will help you to be clear in your own mind precisely what you aim to achieve. If you are not absolutely sure about your specific goal, then you will lay yourself open to being manoeuvred into accepting an outcome that you don't really want.

Keep notes

Keeping notes provides you with a means of reference so that you can easily recall specific dates, past correspondence, the nature and contents of discussions and phone calls that you have had with various officials. This adds tremendous strength to your argument when fighting someone's corner. With all its rules, regulations and red tape, bureaucracy can be thrown into disarray by people who are able to quote chapter and verse on what has actually taken place. It is always worth following up a meeting, telephone call or conversation with a letter confirming what has been agreed, and of course it is essential that you keep a copy in your file.

Enlist the help of others

Jot down in your file what information you need and where you might be able to get it. You will have to be prepared to do a lot of your own research, and in this respect the Citizens' Advice Bureau and the local library can be invaluable. Don't expect to solve all your problems on your own. If you start to feel despondent and the problem seems as though it has become an unclimbable mountain, then get in touch with friends, voluntary groups and other supporters and between you make a list of all the resources and help that you can identify. Be as creative as possible and approach as many people as you can who will listen, give you the benefit of their thoughts on how you might overcome the problem and perhaps even actively support you. These don't have to be people who know much about learning difficulties. It is amazing how many problems can be overcome by suggestions from people who have no specific knowledge of the matter but can provide some effective answers simply by applying their own skills and experiences from totally unrelated fields.

Prepare your case

Before you make contact, take a leaf out of the Boy Scouts' manual and 'be prepared'. Write down all the arguments you can think of which support your case, and get as many people to help you as you can. Then write down all the arguments which you think people will use to oppose your case. Finally, write down all the counter-arguments you can think of to demolish their objections.

Present your case

In presenting your case you will need to establish your credibility. So try not to show any frustration you may feel by venting your spleen on the person you are seeking to win over—it is vital for you to keep control of the situation. Spiking sarcasm, angry outbursts and negative body language will merely serve to alienate the person who could perhaps be of most help to you. If you are positive and constructive throughout it will be more difficult for people to offer any real resistance. Acknowledging what they have accomplished so far, and showing your appreciation of the achievements of which you approve, is a good opening gambit. This will make them well disposed towards you and what you are trying to do. Then, if you do need to express some dissatisfaction, it is more likely to be received in a positive light.

Whatever you do, stick to the point. It is all too easy to be sidetracked onto other issues and to end up spending the entire meeting talking about matters which are of no particular relevance to your own situation. If necessary, you will have to keep on coming back to the subject you have come to discuss. Sound like an old broken record if you must, but don't lose sight of your reason for being there in the first place.

Don't be surprised if professionals try to put you down. Remember, no matter how nicely you may put it, there will be those bureaucrats for whom you will be posing problems, who will see you as a nuisance. Therefore, you may well be hit with phrases like 'That's rather unreasonable you know,' or 'Don't you think you're being unrealistic?' or 'I wouldn't have thought that was what most caring parents would want for their child,' and so on. It will pay you to refrain from rising to the bait; simply respond by saying something like, 'I understand what you are saying, but . . .' and then continue, unruffled, with the issue that is concerning you.

Often professionals will use their own jargon, either without realising that some of the words and phrases they use will be unfamiliar to others, or as a deliberate ploy to keep you at a disadvantage and to impress you with their status as an expert so that you will not be tempted to challenge them. Whenever jargon is used, and for whatever reason, if you are unable to understand fully what they mean, don't hesitate to ask for plain language to be used. This is in no way an admission of your ignorance but more a reflection on their professionalism and inability to communicate. At the end of the day, fancy labels and phrases usually turn out to be just pious ways of describing very down-to-earth conditions and practices.

Finally, when you are negotiating your position, it is as well to refer to both sides of the issue, giving your own viewpoint more weight, of course. This will show that you have thought it through and that you have fully comprehended all the aspects. This way no one can say that you have not understood the situation or that you are being unreasonable.

OVERCOMING INTIMIDATION

Whether intentionally or not, professionals can be very intimidating and you may have to find ways of overcoming your own feelings of uncertainty or inadequacy. I was once told that if I was being made to feel inferior, I should try to imagine the other person performing everyday functions that we all have to carry out, like shaving, cutting toenails or sitting on the lavatory, perhaps. It is not always a pleasant image to conjure up, but it does seem to do away with that air of grandeur and help you to see yourself in a more equal light.

It is always worth taking a close friend along with you so that he or she can help you to recall events afterwards, share in the experience and give you extra support. Sometimes it is even worth taking someone whom you don't know very well but who looks the part. This could be someone wearing a suit and toting an expensive-looking briefcase. You simply introduce this ally as 'a friend' and he or she will take copious notes while the officials are speaking, every so often interrupting to ask the speaker if he or she would repeat the last sentence, and then making a big play of taking it down word for word. This can be most disconcerting for professionals and will actually begin to turn the tables of intimidation against them. They will assume that your 'friend' is in some way very professionally or perhaps legally qualified, when in fact he or she may be a plumber or your local greengrocer!

GET THE MOST OUT OF FORMAL MEETINGS

Before you attend a meeting, write down the important questions you want to ask, and if at the meeting you are unable to obtain the answers there and then, ask the chairperson or someone else to undertake to find out the answers for you. Don't forget to take his name and telephone number so that you can chase him up if the information is not forthcoming within a reasonable time. Also, remember to follow up the meeting with a letter confirming what has been said and agreed. If minutes are being taken, then of course you need not write a follow-up letter, but you should ensure that you will be sent a copy. When you receive it, read it through carefully and, if there are any inaccurate statements, write immediately and ask for them to be amended.

A strange thing about professionals is their system of career advancement. Take the teaching profession as an example. Class teachers work directly with children every day and as such have more effect upon the children they teach than anyone else in the education system. The more experienced and effective the teacher becomes, the more she is promoted into situations quite remote from children and what she does best. Finally, when she reaches the pinnacle of advancement and becomes Director of Education, the time she spends with individual pupils is a mere fraction of her responsibilities and she may be in serious danger of losing touch with the sharp end of her business—indeed, in some cases, whether they realise it or not, the important individuality of children may be lost in their overall pupil population and statistics until they are eventually seen as little more than a commodity. For this reason it is often a good idea to include your son or daughter in any meetings, to remind people that they are discussing a human being and that any decisions made will have a considerable effect on his or her life. If this is not possible, then a short video (not more than ten minutes) or at least a photograph can be taken along and shown to those present.

Form a network of support

If you are going to speak up for people who themselves have difficulty being heard, then they will be dependent upon your commitment and ability to ensure that their best interests are being considered and met. You yourself will need to develop a network of friends and supporters to help you deal with those times of depression and sheer fatigue that you are going to face now and then, because it is most unlikely that all will run smoothly. However you may be feeling inside, when negotiating your case you will do well to present a balanced and controlled exterior. Do your best to be in possession of all the facts, think out the arguments against you beforehand and plan your counter-arguments. If at any time you feel that the meeting is getting out of your control or going against you, explain that you feel too upset to continue and call for an adjournment.

At all times remember that you are closest to the person whom you are representing, and in that respect you are more in touch with his or her needs than anyone else. No matter how experienced or well qualified they may say they are, at best their experience and qualifications will apply to the field of learning difficulties in general, whilst yours will be concentrated on one person in particular. Whatever you do, no matter how tired you become or how downtrodden you may feel, if you believe you are right and that it is in the best interests of the person you are supporting, NEVER GIVE UP! Remember, if enough people hit their heads against a brick wall—it will fall down.

Some places where you can get help

Community Health Council. Every area has one. The address can be found in the telephone book.

Citizen's Advice Bureau (CAB). Look up the telephone directory for your local area.

Welfare Rights. The address of your nearest office can be obtained from the local library or your Citizens' Advice Bureau.

Values Into Action. Can provide you with information and other contacts regarding matters concerning people who have learning disabilities. Their address is in the listing at the end of this book.

Passport Parents Group. A small group of parents based in the North-West who have had considerable success in gaining supported places in mainstream schools for children who have severe learning difficulties. Their address can also be found at the end of this book.

MIND (National Association for Mental Health). Are always very helpful with support and information. Their head office is at 22 Harley Street, London W1N 2ED. Tel: 071–637–0741.

Elected Representatives. The name and address of your local councillors and Members of Parliament can be obtained from your library or Citizen's Advice Bureau.

The Disability Rights Handbook. Published each year and has a great deal of valuable information for those who have a disability and their families. It is produced by The Disability Alliance ERA at First Floor Flat East, Universal House, 88–94 Wentworth Street, London E1 7SA. Tel: (for advice) 071–247 8763; (for administration) 071–247 8776. Can be contacted between 11 a.m. and 3 p.m. Monday to Friday.

The Centre for Studies on Integration in Education. Provides support and up-to-date information for those seeking to gain a place in mainstream education for a child who has additional needs. The address is at the end of this book.

8 Living with Adolescence—'That Difficult Age'

> 'When you are a baby, you can see your mummy's bosom, but when you grow up it's not allowed and I think that's a silly rule.'
> Vivienne, aged six years

I don't know about you, but the word 'adolescent' has just about the same appeal for me as do 'Poll Tax' or 'politician'. Somewhere along the road it has gathered a bad press and I don't find myself readily warming to it. Some people refer to it as 'that difficult age', but the truth is that, in childhood (and as adults, come to that), we pass through more than just one 'difficult age'. In fact, when I think about it, throughout my life people have *always* seemed to refer to *me* as being at 'that difficult age'. I first remember it when I was about five, although my parents would probably say that I had been through several difficult phases before that. But as a boy of four or five, just about every sentence I spoke seemed to begin infuriatingly with the word 'why' and was punctuated with a screwed-up face, portraying gross confusion. Added to this, it was invariably delivered with a high-frequency whine in my voice, which was guaranteed to drive all those adults who were on the receiving end to screaming pitch. What's more, my questions were virtually impossible for any parent to answer satisfactorily, unless of course, he or she happened to be a competent physicist, philosopher, ordained priest, celebrated legal eagle and Nobel Prize-winning biologist all rolled into one.

'Dad, why can't dogs talk?'

'Mum, why do you say that *you're* cold and then tell *me* to put *my* coat on?'

'Are there Easter eggs in heaven?'

'If God is everywhere, Mum, why do we have to go to church?'

'Dad, does the Queen have to go to the toilet just like us?' . . . and so on into horrendous infinity.

Then came those adolescent years, when my body suddenly began to take on an unfamiliar life of its own. At this age I was somewhat unnerved to discover hair sprouting with great gusto from a variety of totally unexpected places and my voice, which had always been a rather boyish soprano, would every now and then lapse alarmingly, mid sentence, into a deep baritone. As if this were not enough, unbeknown to me my hormones which, I may say, had always been quite orderly and well-behaved until then, began to take on the characteristics of a firework display, causing me considerable emotional chaos without my really understanding why. I couldn't be sure if I had achieved manhood at last or was still a boy.

After a while it became apparent that I was neither. Instead people called me a 'youth' or, even worse, a 'teenager', the latter usually uttered through clenched teeth. A youth, it seemed, was someone who had reached that in-between age, someone who was destined, for a while at least, to remain in such a state of confusion as to go through life holding a comic in one hand and a cigarette in the other—too old to act childish and too young to be considered a grown-up.

When I reached the end of my school life, although still in a condition of adolescence, I had made it by then to a somewhat comparatively privileged position. Being in the sixth form I was among the eldest in the school and this, I was given to understand, entitled me to some measure of respect which, up until then, as a mere school boy, had largely escaped me. Overnight I was made a prefect (or a *perfect*, as some uncharitable children sneeringly called us) and a member of the school council to boot. For this I was afforded certain courtesies and a degree of trust. Even teachers (that almost holy form of life) encouraged my independence and allowed me free periods when I was left to study by myself. It was a rude awakening, therefore, when I finished school and started work, only to find that my standing in the world had all been turned upon its head again, in one fell swoop. Suddenly I was very much the junior once more, a species who had it all to learn and could not be relied upon to carry out even the simplest task without it being properly checked. My status, such as it was, crashed instantly from one of privilege and esteem to one of general dogsbody.

Since then, amongst other things, I have ventured through life in the shape of a husband, a father, an employer, an employee, a house-owner, a tenant, a voter and a tax-payer. As a father, I have watched my own two children go through the same obstacle course of 'difficult ages' that I once clambered over, but from an entirely different perspective. Looking back, I realise that all of us have been through the experience of adolescence in much the same way and I don't have any reason to suppose that, if the label 'learning difficulties' had been attached to me, I would have experienced the turmoil of puberty in any significantly different way.

Nevertheless, when we are confronted with the effects of adolescence in a youngster who has learning difficulties, we can become quite unnerved and get things out of all proportion. Rapid hormone growth and disability can suddenly seem like a recipe for panic. Before we know it we have developed a distinct tendency to focus upon phrases like 'challenging behaviour' and 'emotional disturbance', rather than considering such things in the light of 'normal' adolescence which we know something about because we have all been through it. Certainly, we have all been a source of anxiety to our parents, and this is the time of life when it is our turn to be the recipients. Insanity, they say, is hereditary—we get it from our children.

On the subject of parenting, my mother once told me that the first ten years are the worst, but I can tell you, it isn't true. Parenting through the teens can be every bit as traumatic for the parents as it is for their children. Keeping a broad perspective, engaging sound common sense, attempting to bridge the generation gap and 'keeping your head when all about you are losing theirs', can seem like a task designed for Superman (or should I say Superperson?). The confusion, in puberty, of not quite knowing whether you are yet an adult or still a child can be further compounded by your parents and other adults around you, if they continually show that they regard you as some sort of eternal child in an adult's body.

Unfortunately, this type of malformed concept, which is so easily developed, can take hold in the early years when your children are young and become quite ingrained in your head and therefore in your attitude, throughout their progress into adulthood. It starts, perhaps, when they are babies and you get concerned that they have not yet learnt how to sit up by themselves when other babies of the same age are already crawling and walking. As time goes by you notice that other children are becoming quite chatty whilst your own child still has not made so much as a dribbly babbling sound. Finally, you are one day told that your son or daughter has a learning difficulty and, from that time on, if you allow it, your expectations of your child may be very low. You find yourself watching other children grow and develop whilst your own seems to grow very well, but not develop.

From this, some people, whether they are parents, teachers, doctors or whatever, make the mistake of assuming that although this child has the same physique as other children of the same age, he is somehow very much younger inside. Of course, his learning difficulties will mean that he has significant developmental delays, but if he is allowed he is still likely to have an interest in the same things as others of his own age. Whether he has additional needs or not, a seventeen-year-old boy will usually want to know about pop music, fashion, cars or motorbikes and seventeen-year-old girls.

The misunderstanding whereby learning difficulties equals eternal child is often created by the notion of mental age. At one time, doctors and psychologists used to (and some still do) use tests in order to convert what the child had scored from a particular test into a mental age. Thus, parents may be told that their nine-year-old has a mental age of, say, eighteen months. As a result there is an understandable tendency for parents to treat their nine-year-old like an eighteen-month-old in every respect and in all situations. This means that their youngster never has much opportunity to become mature in any way other than physically. Some parents actually prefer their maturing son or daughter to remain childlike in his or her teens and adulthood. After all, the younger years are the best for some parents who enjoy their child's dependence; at the same time, such an attitude avoids, or so they think, the complications of the child becoming a sexual being and makes it easier to keep him or her safe from the wicked world.

Growing up under these conditions means that such children will simply learn how to be helpless and highly dependent, while their parents are destined to go through life getting older and less able to cope, but having to respond to the needs of their bigger and heavier son or daughter. Where this situation has prevailed throughout their childhood, we see men and women in their twenties, thirties, forties and older, still grasping teddy bears, wearing clothes which are entirely inappropriate to their age, acting coy and shy, cuddling up to mummy and exhibiting a whole range of other similar behaviours which we would expect from a child rather than an adult.

For most children, we have an expectation that they will eventually become independent, self-determining and a person in their own right, but as soon as the two magic words 'learning difficulty' are uttered, we somehow tend to let our overprotective instincts take over and succeed only in 'smothering' rather than mothering our child. During the in-between years, whether we have learning difficulties or not, there are some considerations in our lives which suddenly start to become particularly important to us, such as our self-identity, our relationships, our acceptance socially, our need to belong, our need to experiment and our vulnerability during this experimentation. As parents of youngsters who have learning disabilities it is essential for us to be in touch with how they might be seeing things and, within the bounds of common sense, afford them some extra space and begin to respect them as emerging adults.

Acknowledging their sexuality

Sex always seems to be regarded as a rather sticky subject, and never more so than when it is applied to people who have a learning difficulty. The fact is that a fulfilled and satisfying sex life, however you may define it, is important for most people and to deny that enjoyment to some, simply because they have failed to obtain a particular score in some IQ test, seems to me to be a direct infringement of the United Nations 1971 General Assembly Declaration of Freedom for People who are Mentally Handicapped. What can be more ludicrous than denying access to a sound sexual relationship on the grounds of some sort of intellectual means test?

Of course, as far as sex is concerned, we have more than just equal opportunity to worry about; we also have to consider our responsibilities towards people with learning disabilities, to ensure that they are well versed in all that a sex life entails. Sex education in some form is essential to anyone who is going to develop a sexual drive and it has to begin well before puberty. This means responding to questions honestly and meaningfully, no matter what the age of your child. It also means responding positively to what you regard as inappropriate sexual behaviour. All children need to know that self-exploration and touching or showing their genitalia is something only done at bath time or in private and not in front of Auntie Jean and Uncle Ben at tea time.

Above all, it is the parents' attitude when dealing with these situations that is of most significance. Embarrassment, or a chastising edge to your voice and actions, will only serve to instil an unhealthy approach to sex in your child's mind and possibly create problems later on. Where your youngster has a learning difficulty which makes verbal communication very hard, distraction with other things or removing him calmly (and not as a punishment) to the bathroom or his bedroom is one way of dealing with public behaviour which he has to understand is only acceptable in private.

Young women need to know about menstruation before they begin their cycles. They should be given some idea of what to expect and the practicalities of coping with their periods. Precisely how this is done will depend upon your daughter's learning disabilities. Sex education is as essential as road sense and it doesn't end with simply knowing where it is all right to masturbate and how to fit a sanitary towel. Contrary to some people's fears, sex education does not act as a detonator which releases a torrent of uncontrollable libido within those who have learning difficulties. On the contrary, failure to equip such people with a practical working knowledge and understanding of their own sexual organs and the complexities of personal relationships will ensure that they remain childlike in their naivete, which will render them defenceless against exploitation. Also, their ignorance of sexual matters could one day lead them quite innocently into trouble with the law.

Sex should not be regarded as a masonic secret, only to be bestowed upon those who have been accepted into the club. Sex is a fact of life and a pretty important one, too, since we each owe our very existence to it and are reliant upon it to safeguard our survival as a species. There can be no justifiable moral argument that favours the denial of sexual rights to people on the grounds of intellectual ability, although those of us who are parentally or professionally involved do have a responsibility to see that the vulnerability of people who have learning disabilities is given some reasonable degree of protection. This needs to be provided in a common-sense way, which means finding a workable balance that avoids the unacceptable restrictions of overprotection and focuses more upon practical guidance and support. Nobody would advocate that parents or staff should 'play God', but some judgements do have to be made regularly, so that the person or people concerned can gain reasonable access appropriate to their age and circumstances, with the minimum of risk to themselves and others.

So what would we consider to be appropriate? The answer, of course, will vary according to individual situations, but there are some broad guidelines to be found in what the public at large nowadays seem to find acceptable. There is also the law which lays down definite parameters about people's sexual behaviour. These can be used as a type of yardstick when attempting to apply some judgement to our own situations. The following are some of the points to bear in mind:

1 These days, safe sex is a must and young people need to understand, in precise practical terms, exactly what that means and how to practise it. They need to know about sexually transmitted diseases and how to avoid them. They therefore also need to know what condoms are and how to use them. They also need to know the safe alternatives to full penetration.
2 Social attitudes have changed radically in recent years. People now have sexual experience at a much younger age than ever before. Sex before marriage is now regarded as the norm and marriage itself appears no longer to be a social necessity.
3 The taboo of masturbation has long since disappeared and the majority of young men and women readily indulge privately for their own sexual pleasure. It is no

longer regarded as harmful or as something to be discouraged.

4 Homosexual relationships ceased to be outlawed some thirty-odd years ago and, in general terms, whilst our society seems to be somewhat divided in its attitudes towards gay people, on the whole there has been a steady move towards greater acceptance of this form of sexual choice.
5 Society also seems to have a mixed view over the issue of soft pornography. Generally it is not illegal, and magazines, videos and so on are easily available in the high street, catering to the tastes of both men and women. There is, however, a wide view that pornography is degrading to women.
6 Hard core pornography is illegal in the United Kingdom although elsewhere cable television channel broadcasts are in operation.
7 A recent survey claimed that one man in ten now uses the services of a prostitute, and the issue of legalising prostitution in this country is officially brought forward for discussion from time to time.
8 Sex chat-lines are also a product of our times and, at the moment at least, operate within the law.
9 Sex shops now operate in most cities and large towns, selling vibrators and what they refer to as 'marital aids'.

These are just some of the indications of how our society appears to view sexual behaviour these days. Your own feelings on the matter will of course be the major influence over what is acceptable and what is unacceptable in your home. However, when you have the responsibility of giving guidance to a youngster who has learning difficulties, your own views will need to be tempered in the context of what society regards as the norm for young people today. Making your own values and beliefs known to your children, and guiding them throughout their childhood, is sound parenting, but attempting to enforce strict standards of sexual conduct when adolescence begins, without regard for what others of their own age are doing around them, is both foolhardy and largely ineffective.

Whether you are the parent of a young person with learning difficulties who lives at home, or a professional who has the day-to-day responsibility for a number of people in a residential service, what to do in practice, about a variety of sexual matters that occur in everyday situations, will seem fraught with dilemmas. In our own lives, generally speaking, we seem mostly to hide our sexual activities. Indulgence in soft porn magazines, videos, masturbation and so on are the sort of things which most people prefer to conceal. Those who have learning difficulties, on the other hand, often show no such inhibitions, and one of the first things they must learn is the need for appropriateness and discretion. Whilst masturbation may now be acknowledged as a perfectly acceptable pastime, it also has to be understood that it is not a good idea to do it in the middle of Sainsbury's.

Within some special services there are staff who feel that it is important actually to teach the art of masturbation to their residents. Whilst I can appreciate the human rights rationale behind this thinking, I have to say that I believe it to be both dangerous and unnecessary. Dangerous, in that a very fine line exists between what is considered to be sex therapy and what constitutes a sexual offence, and unnecessary because sexual arousal hardly needs to be taught. I cannot think of a single person of my acquaintance who has had to take a course in how to instigate sexual relief. You really do not need a PhD in order to scratch an itch. Hunger and sexual appetite are primary drives and, as such, require little or no instruction in how to take reactionary measures.

Theory, of course, is nearly always rather different from practice. Whilst we may find it relatively easy to declare ourselves in favour of extending to people who have learning difficulties the same sexual freedom that we all seem to enjoy, it can nevertheless turn into a somewhat hollow gesture once we discover what it really means. Our own sexual hang-ups can prevent us from allowing others access to a sex life which is meaningful to them, for whilst sex is enjoyable, it can also be a major source of anxiety. We may consider ourselves sexually confident and well-adjusted, but this doesn't seem to stop us from thumbing vigorously through documents like the latest Kinsey Report that may come our way, in order to see if our own sexual performance measures up to the national average. Sex is a complex business and appetites and individual tastes vary enormously. Psychologists should beware, for there is no standard to measure here, nor any definite norm. All that exists is a range of individual preferences.

Looking around the so-called ordinary people in our society, we find them to be made up of heterosexuals, homosexuals, bisexuals, lesbians, cross-dressers, transvestites and fetishists. Within the constraints of the law they can each follow their own selected form of sexual pleasure in the privacy of their own home and with other consenting adults. It is reasonable to assume, then, that those who have learning difficulties will also be made up of a similar mixture of heterosexuals, homosexuals, bisexuals and so on. Why, then, do some of us seek to confine their choice of sexual expression? It is done of course, in the name of protection, which at the end of the day simply serves further to limit the lives that they lead. Balanced against this we have a responsibility to safeguard their interests, and now, more than ever, staff of residential establishments desperately need some guidelines that truly address the issues in practical terms and allow them to decide and agree where the boundaries lie.

Whether they live at home or within a residential service, people who have learning difficulties do not just need approval from parents and professionals to have access to sexual experience, they also need to be allowed the time, place and opportunities. Often, so much of their waking life seems to be supervised. A simple act like taking a long, luxurious bath can rarely be enjoyed without interruption from someone who feels it important to keep checking up on them. Privacy comes at a premium for people who have learning difficulties, who continually seem to find themselves 'policed' by one adult or another. The ideal attitude to adopt is one which is accepting of sexual behaviour as opposed to encouraging. Knocking on the door and then waiting to be invited in is a common courtesy which we extend to most people, so why not those who have additional needs? Adolescent sexual exploration may sometimes be embarrassing, but it is a normal phase of our development. Why, then, should we regard it as anything but normal for those who have learning difficulties? In one situation we accept it, in the other we reach for referral forms and behaviour modification programmes.

For years, people who have learning disabilities have had their rights denied, their feelings disregarded and, on many an occasion, have become the victims of 'legal abuse'. Some people find it difficult to understand why anyone who has a low intellectual ability should seek a sexual relationship, enter into marriage or a permanent partnership and want to have a family. Why should this be so incredible? After all, it seems to be what most of the rest of us do, and not always very successfully. But the very thought of a woman who has learning disabilities becoming pregnant is, for some, one of the worst catastrophes that can befall them.

Our key responsibility is to ensure that those who have learning difficulties are properly supported so that they can become as independent as possible and have the opportunity to live a full life. Giving and receiving a commitment to a partner and bringing up a family are, for some, part and parcel of living a full life, so why should we seek to prevent it? It is certainly not unheard of for couples who have learning difficulties successfully to bring up their own children, with appropriate assistance. In fact, in many instances they do a far better job than some so-called 'normal' couples whose treatment of their children can be much less than caring.

Even so, sterilisation, abortion and social service care orders all too often seem to be the first line of defence imposed on expectant mothers who have learning difficulties. In one residential service that I came across, a hysterectomy was the prerequisite for any young woman of eighteen or over who sought admission there. Where a fear of unwanted pregnancy exists, the law now provides women who have learning difficulties with clear rights when it comes to sterilisation. Since they are regarded as being incapable of granting consent for themselves, such drastic measures can no longer be taken simply for the benefit of staff or parents. All other forms of contraception must now first be considered. A prospect of child-bearing must exist and action can only be taken if there are good health reasons and the operation conforms to sound health practice.

Whilst these rights do exist, I have to say that women who have learning disabilities still usually have their new-born babies taken into care and are rendered incapable of having any more children, often never understanding why. In any event, when it comes to people who have learning disabilities, the law, as they say, is an ass. In legal terms, such people are still referred to as 'defectives'. A defective, says the 1983 Mental Health Act, is a person who has 'a state of arrested or incomplete development of mind, which includes severe impairment of intelligence and social functioning'. The law regards people like this as being incapable of giving their consent, and so anyone who has sexual relations with them is automatically having unlawful sexual intercourse. However, the law does not prevent a person who has learning difficulties from entering into the state of matrimony. Just like anyone else, no parental consent is required over the age of eighteen. In legal terms, though, if they consummate their marriage, under the 1983 Mental Health Act they have, it seems, committed an offence. In practice, wide discretion is afforded to the police in situations like this, but it does give some idea of what people with learning difficulties are up against in establishing equal rights within a legal system which regards them as defective.

People who have learning disabilities need just what we all need: a sound education and information about sexual matters; to know how their own body works and what it is designed to do; to have access to safe sexual experience. They need opportunities to meet and choose partners, to know how to present themselves through good standards of hygiene and self-care, to become skilled in applying make-up, grooming and in developing a sense of style in the clothes they wear. They need access to contraception and they need their personalities and sexuality to be recognised.

Acknowledging their need for space and a good self-image

If you have been successful in avoiding those 'special' institutions for your child in the earlier years, then no doubt he or she will have shared her time with local children of her own age, rather than with other disabled children whom she only ever saw at the special school. She will therefore have friends with whom she has grown up over a period of years. She will have been involved in all the usual events and interests enjoyed by other children of her age and locality. As a teenager, like her friends, she will now want to stay out later, go to parties, use make-up, wear fashionable hair styles and clothes, smoke and drink and do all the things we once did but dread our own children doing. This, I suppose, is where the sleepless nights begin.

There is a vast difference between guidance and direction and, on the whole, guidance is more likely to be your salvation as a parent than the authoritarian and dictatorial attitude of direction. Remember, in the years of adolescence much will depend on the sound foundation that you have built with your child during the earlier years. Your son's or daughter's need for independence does not only become apparent in the teens, but is in fact a continuous process from birth. If you have been reassuring and have encouraged your child to do all the smaller tasks for herself when she was younger, then not only will she have the confidence to tackle bigger challenges, but you too will have developed that very necessary ability to let go a little. In the teenage years, that element of trust between parent and child becomes all-important. Where learning difficulties are concerned, parents have to find ways of realistically assessing their youngster's ability in given situations, calculate the risk and decide what they will allow as a responsible parent. These decisions can be made based on the following:

1 *Having some trust in their friends.* When your child has grown up with friends who themselves do not have a learning disability, an element of responsibility is likely to have established itself in the relationship. As a parent you will have had an opportunity to witness this, and your confidence in their reliability will have also been growing. Allowing your son's or daughter's friends to take him or her to school without you for the first time will have been every bit as traumatic as seeing them go to the pictures together or dancing at the disco for the first time. You may want to build in your own safeguards at a discreet distance without their knowledge for the first few times, but however you appease your own anxieties, it is necessary to allow some freedom.
2 *Make-up.* Take into account what is generally regarded as being acceptable for young people these days. At what age are their friends allowed to wear make-up? What sort of make-up is now regarded as trendy, and in what circumstances? For instance, many an older woman would have a blue fit at seeing some of the colours of lipstick that are worn these days.
3 *Coming home time and bedtime.* These arrangements, too, should have some parity with those of their friends of the same age. Times need to be agreed beforehand and they should understand what the consequences will be if they abuse your trust by coming in late—for

instance, being grounded for a week. Watches that bleep to a pre-set time are quite cheap and can be effective as a reminder for those who are unable to read the time.

4 *Smoking and drinking.* Most youngsters seem to want to experiment in this area at some time, so if it is going to be done at all, then it is far better for it to be done at home and in your presence where you can have some control.

5 *Income.* What they receive in the way of pocket money should be earned in some way, from having the responsibility of jobs around the house, geared to their ability. The amount will also need to correspond with what others of their age receive. Learning the value of money can only be done when you are expected to earn it and allowed to suffer the consequences of managing your own budget.

6 *Youth gangs.* These can be a by-product of adolescence, and although they are in one sense a normal phenomenon, they are hardly the sort of thing that any parent would want to see their son or daughter heavily engaged in. Having learning disabilities means that you can be easily led and so find yourself involved in criminal offences, drug abuse, acid parties, raves, solvent abuse and all the worst scenarios that we can imagine for our youngsters. It goes without saying, therefore, that you will need to check up inconspicuously but regularly, on the company your child is keeping. Never, during their teen years, get too complacent. As a parent it will always be your responsibility to know where they are going, what they are going for and who they will be with.

When it comes to adolescence, a parent's place is always in the wrong—or so it will often seem. The fact that your son or daughter has learning disabilities will not exempt him or her from going through the long helter-skelter of trials and tribulations that we associate with bouncing hormones. Mood swings, loss of temper, self-assertion, insecurity, are just a few of the features that we have all experienced in our teens and have now mostly forgotten. They are the characteristics of adolescence, not mental handicap, and are shared by all youngsters who are at that time of life when they are beginning to leave their childhood behind and are becoming young men and women. Whatever your child's ability, no matter how severe his learning difficulties may be, he is entitled to grow up like everyone else. Attempting to keep him as a child forever will not protect him from the outside world, it will only fail to equip him with ways of dealing with it. Parents may feel that it is much simpler and safer to keep their child as a child, for them it may be true, but for their youngster it amounts to nothing more than a grave disservice. Adulthood is not something that is awarded according to intelligence. If that were the case, then half our Cabinet would still be toddlers. Adulthood is achieved through maturation, and each of us, as parents, has a significant role to play in guiding our children through all the difficult stages.

9 Together We Are Better—Forming an Effective Parent Group

'Never doubt that a small group of people can change the world. Indeed, it is the only thing that ever has.' Margaret Mead

Supporting your son or daughter in taking all the opportunities to get as much out of their life as he or she can will in turn mean that you yourself are going to need a good deal of support. Sometimes making alliances with other people who share your predicament is a good way of gaining from each other's strengths and experiences and is likely to enable everyone to generate fresh ideas, develop some confidence and, in general, provide an atmosphere of good morale. Joining one of the established large charitable organisations is one way of doing this and can certainly give you much-needed information. Being part of a large organisation also means that you can access some clout, which can sometimes be mobilised nationally, if need be.

However, many parents find that they only attend this type of meeting once or twice and then drop out. This happens when they find that much of the evening is spent debating who will be running which stall at their local fête, rather than discussing some of the key issues that concern them. Unfortunately, as you may well find, some parents' organisations can lose their way and end up as a collection of people busying themselves with things like tea rotas and raffles, rather than supporting each other to further the cause that first brought them together. There are always tell-tale signs that will indicate to some extent what sort of group you are faced with. You will need to make your own assessment of its usefulness, so when you first go, the way in which you are treated as a newcomer will be all-revealing.

You may find, for instance, that you are approached by a person who introduces herself as the secretary rather than by her first name. Many voluntary groups are plagued with such people who want to portray themselves as some sort of para-professional. What they seek is a certain status for themselves, and they are usually about as much help to you as a chocolate teapot. You will recognise them immediately: they will be the ones armed with a clipboard and with a biro attached to a cord hung round their necks. They will have one of those formal fixed smiles that disappear as quickly as they came. Most of their dialogue with you will be about the cost of membership and the rules of the organisation, rather than asking how you are managing and how they can help. If most of the members of your local group are like this, then I would suggest that it is time for you to start your own informal but effective parent group.

Sadly, some long-established organisations may be run by ageing parents who have become quite inflexible in their thinking and are intolerant of younger parents who seem to them to want more for their sons and daughters than they think they should have. There can be an obvious division in some groups where confrontation occurs between the older parents who had no support when they were young, and consequently were forced to use the institutions which were all that was offered to them in those days, and the younger mums and dads who expect more from the services today. Sometimes, resentment that the younger parents are seemingly having all the help which they themselves once needed is displayed in their vigorous support for more residential institutions for people with learning disabilities and rejection of the community care initiatives. There is little point in joining organisations like this in the hope that you will change them or make them see reason. Their heavy emotional investment over the years makes it almost impossible for them to take a different position.

Starting your own group, or joining one that someone else is starting, can be a great source of comfort to you, as well as creating some positive energy which can have a galvanising effect on all concerned. Just chatting with a few like-minded people over coffee is a good way to start. Once people begin to empathise with each other, it is not long before they are sharing confidences and anxieties which bond them. Meet whenever and wherever you like; formalising things need only happen when and if you choose. Ask people along to talk to your group, even if there are only half-a-dozen of you. Don't just invite people from special services: ask those who are in the mainstream, too, and see how they feel about disability and having people who have learning difficulties using their services. Most of them may not have thought much about it until you asked them. They could turn out to be strong advocates for you, either now or at some time in the future.

Formalising your group

As time goes on you may feel that, together, you want to take action on some of the aims you have been discussing. You may want to start writing to individuals or organisations as a group, or perhaps you need to apply for a grant of some sort in order to get an idea put into practice. Whatever it may be, there could come a time when you will need to organise yourselves a little more formally than you have before. First you will need to be clear about what you want to achieve. Do you want to become more systematic to fulfil one particular project, or are your aims much broader? Do you want to achieve something which has a limited life-span, or are you in for the long haul? Is there a particular activity that you want to do straight away? Are there other things that you will want to accomplish at a later date? All these questions are for discussion in your group so that, right from the start, you can achieve some consensus on your specific aims and goals.

Taking yourselves through the PATH procedure described in Chapter Six is an excellent way to pull your group together and focus upon those things which are important to you. Write down a few short sentences that sum up your aims and objectives and discuss them with each other until you are agreed that these words declare exactly what you as a group are about.

Once your goals have been clearly defined, you will need to put together a formal organisational structure. Don't be put off by all this formality; it can be fun and a way of achieving the things that your son or daughter badly needs. Organisations of this kind need a chairperson, whose role it is to see that the group keeps on track and that things run as smoothly as possible. You will need a secretary to deal with all the correspondence for the group, to let everyone know what correspondence has been received and to write the replies according to the wishes of the group. Then, of course, there is the treasurer. This person does not have to be a great mathematician, just someone who can keep an account of what money is collected and spent. If you can manage housekeeping budgets, then you can do the job of a treasurer. Depending upon how many of you there are, you may also need to have a committee to carry out the transactions of your group.

These matters can all be decided as you design your group's constitution. A constitution is simply a name for the rules and regulations which you all agree upon for your organisation. For example, who can vote on issues? What is the least number (quorum) that can hold an official meeting? Will members have to pay an annual subscription—if so, how much? You can easily obtain specimen copies of constitutions for local groups and adapt it to your own needs from:

National Federation of Community Organisations, 8, Upper Street, LONDON N1 OPQ.

or from:
Civic Trust, 17, Carlton House Terrace, LONDON SW1Y 5AW.

If approached in the right way, a friendly solicitor may well help you to draft your constitution without charging. Don't be afraid to ask—he can only say no, in which case he will probably feel a lot meaner than you will by doing it.

One of the first things you will have to decide in drafting your constitution is what name to call yourselves. Remember, when choosing a name, it should reflect your concerns whilst at the same time preserving the dignity of those for whom it is to operate. On the whole, it is advisable to avoid creating a logo for yourselves, as it so often proves difficult to get a design which portrays the right message. Whilst you may be very clear in your own minds what your logo represents, other people outside your group may read it in an entirely different way. You will also need a dissolution clause, which states clearly what will happen to any remaining assets should your organisation cease to exist. When you start a formal organisation, you need to think beforehand about the eventuality of it closing, just as when you buy a house, you need to think about how easily it might sell should you want to dispose of it in the future. There are several ways in which you can set yourselves up, some of which are listed below.

AS AN ASSOCIATION, SOCIETY OR CLUB

These organisations are run by a committee of elected members and are among the simplest of the organisational structures. The problem with an association, society or club is that it cannot itself own property which has to be put in the name of trustees. Officers of this sort of organisation are in fact personally liable in law for what goes on in the association and will also have to fork out, should their organisation not have enough assets to meet its financial responsibilities.

AS A TRUST

This is run by a group of people known as 'trustees' who are responsible for seeing that the organisation administers its funds in accordance with its stated aims and objectives. Whilst the trust itself can hold property, the trustees still have personal responsibility in law.

AS A COMPANY LIMITED BY GUARANTEE

Whilst it is more expensive to set up a company, it does mean that the directors have no personal liability in the event of it running into financial difficulties. Directors are elected by the membership and have a responsibility to see that things are carried out in accordance with the aims and objectives of the organisation. Although it has corporate status, unlike other companies it is limited not by share capital but by guarantee, and as such it has no shares and cannot distribute any profits to its members. Companies limited by guarantee come under the jurisdiction of the Companies Act and have to file properly audited accounts each year at Companies House.

AS A REGISTERED CHARITY

Several benefits result from becoming a registered charity, among which is the fact that many much larger registered charities will only provide you with grants or donations if you have registered status yourself. The Charity Commission is the regulating body and all applications must be made to it. Your accounts will have to be properly audited and sent to it each year and are open to public scrutiny. The process of becoming registered is notoriously slow but well worth the effort. Officers of the Charity Commission will want to see that you have a properly constituted organisation and will pay particular attention to your organisation's objectives to assure themselves that they are charitable in law. Some of the key phrases used, which are considered to be legally charitable, are things like:

- Relief of poverty and distress

- Promotion of health and welfare
- Advancement of religion
- Promotion of the arts
- Promotion of research
- Advancement of education

Once you are registered as a charity, your organisation will be entitled to tax benefits. Moreover other people will see it as a 'legitimate organisation' which will make fund-raising that little bit easier. However, there can be disadvantages too, depending what you wish to do. Registered charities cannot, for example, undertake political activity, although what is meant by 'political' is unclear as things stand. A number of registered charities seem to lobby quite effectively without any problems. Charities cannot operate as a commercial enterprise, although again, there is nothing to stop you provided you also form a trading company that is limited by guarantee.

For further information about becoming a registered charity contact one of the following:

Register of Charities, Charity Commission, St. Alban's House, 57–60, Haymarket, London SW1Y 4QY.

Register of Charities, Charity Commission, The Deane, Tangier, Taunton TA1 4AY.

Register of Charities, Charity Commission, Graeme House, Derby Square, Liverpool L2.

Keeping a record of your meetings

In formal meetings it is useful beforehand to send members a list of points for discussion. This agenda is usually put together by the chairperson and anyone can ask to have a particular topic or issue included. Having assembled the items in some order, the agenda is sent out to all members by the secretary within a reasonable time before the meeting is due to take place. The secretary also takes notes during the meeting and writes down who is present and what has been agreed by them. These minutes are then sent out to all members with the agenda of the next meeting. An agenda may look something like the example given below:

EAST POPPLEWELL PARENTS GROUP

Next Meeting: 7.30pm – At 29, Action Avenue, East Popplewell

AGENDA

1 To read and approve the minutes of the last meeting (attached).
2 To read out and discuss any correspondence received.
3 Treasurer's report.
4 To discuss becoming a registered charity.
5 To discuss which speaker (and on what topic) to invite to our next meeting.
6 To discuss what opportunities and support can be explored for those who have children with additional needs in the forthcoming school holiday.
7 To discuss supported employment.
8 Time, date and place of next meeting.

Opening your organisation's bank account

Even if you have no money to put in it, a bank account for your group is a matter that will need to be addressed in anticipation of the time when you are presented with your first cheque. Bank charges these days can be quite prohibitive, so you will need to seek out a bank manager who is sympathetic to your cause and will be prepared to waive any charges. In this respect, it is a good idea to think about people you know who could approach a bank on your behalf—someone who does a lot of business with them, perhaps, such as a company director, or someone who has connections with an organisation like the local rotary club. There are some banks which, on a complimentary basis, will actually provide you with someone from their staff to become your treasurer, or at least keep an eye on the way you are keeping your accounts. If you would like this to happen don't be reluctant to make the invitation. If you don't ask, you certainly won't get.

To open your bank account you will have to complete a bank mandate, which is a simple form that asks for a few details and specimen signatures of those who will be authorised by your group to sign cheques. It is always a good idea to have a system requiring two signatures. These could be any two officers of your organisation, such as your chairperson, treasurer, secretary and so on. As your account grows you will want to open a deposit account or find ways of investing your income so that it takes full advantage of any higher rates of interest that you may be able to collect.

No doubt you will have to consider keeping some petty cash available and account for it separately. In this case, be sure to keep any incoming money separate rather than paying it directly into petty cash. That way you will always be able to show on paper exactly where it went and what has happened to it. Make certain, too, that you give and get receipts for every transaction so that everything is properly recorded. If receipts are not readily available, simply make a note of the reason for the expenditure and keep it in your accounts. It makes good sense to keep all petty cash in a special lockable container so that it can never be confused with any of your own money.

Your accounts will need to be audited every year, so right from the start try to find an accountant who would be prepared to do this without charge. Ask other organisations for a name or an introduction. If you really get stuck, contact the Institute of Chartered Accountants in England and Wales, PO Box 433, Moorgate Place, London EC2. This organisation has an up-to-date list of accountants who are prepared to offer their services to charitable organisations without making any charges.

Setting yourselves targets

In order to be successful as a group in achieving your aims and objectives, it is important to give yourselves clear targets and goals. Start from where you want to be and work backwards. As a group, write down precisely what you want to achieve and by when. All you have to remember is that your goals must be both positive and possible. You may decide, for example, that you want to support three members of your group in getting their children into their local mainstream schools in eight months' time. Write down the names of each of the children, the names of the schools that you want them to go to and the actual deadline date by which it is to happen. For example.

Tommy Jones to attend Burbank Primary School by 4 September 1994.
Julia Brown to attend Leafy Lane Infants School by 4 September 1994.
Mandy Smith to attend Fir Tree Primary School by 4 September 1994.

Having decided upon specific goals, you then need to work backwards and plan where you want to be in August 1994, July 1994, June 1994, May 1994 and so on. Finally work out the first step that you are going to take after your meeting has finished. Who will be doing what exactly? If you need to raise money, then plan for it in the same way. How much will you need and by when? If, for example, you will need to raise £4,000 in the next twelve months, record it in a way that breaks it down into feasible steps that you can take to achieve your target. To give an example, Figure 15 shows how much a group has decided to raise each month up to the target date. In January the members have allowed themselves some time to plan and organise events which start

JAN	FEB	MAR	APR	MAY	JUN	JUL	AUG	SEP	OCT	NOV	DEC
NIL	£200	£350	£350	£350	£350	£500	£500	£500	£300	£300	£300

Figure 15. *Defining targets.*

from February. In February they aim to raise £200, so they will have to decide ways in which they might do that. They will have to plan fund-raising events for February, estimate how much each event might raise and decide who is going to be responsible for each event. The planning for February, therefore, might look something like this:

Joan Grey	Give a talk to two local groups: Towns Women's Guild Women's Institute	estimated income £50
Jim Hall	Organise a Barn Dance in the local school	estimated income £100
Maggie Black	Organise a coffee morning at her home	estimated income £20
Kevin Phillips	Organise a quiz at his local pub	estimated income £30

So in January this group will plan all its fund-raising activities for the whole of the coming year. In the meantime, of course, it will also be writing to a range of other organisations applying for grants and donations. It is certainly not unusual for other sponsors to assist you by making the whole sum of £4,000 and more available to you in the form of a donation. However, you will have to put together a sound application if you are to achieve this.

Applying for grants and donations

Central government departments, your Local Authority, grant-making trusts and commercial companies are all potential sources of income, some of them quite considerable. The Wellcome Trust, for example, donates something like £50,000,000 every year. The Directory of Social Change, in its publication *A Guide to the Major Trusts*, gives details of no less than 62 organisations that each regularly gives away over one million pounds every year. It goes on to list a further two hundred and thirty-six that each donates between £100,000 and £993,000, and another 67 that each gives between £10,000 and £99,000 to what they consider to be deserving causes. That is merely one publication; there are of course many others. The Charities Aid Foundation, for instance, goes to print every two years with a book called *Directory of Grant-Making Trusts*. This gives details of the names, addresses, policies and resources of over 2,500 grant-making bodies with a total income of £787,000,000 between them. If you can't afford to buy it, then you will find that most public libraries have a copy in their reference section.

In terms of financial help, then, there seems to be no shortage; you simply have to present a clear and convincing case. Make sure that you do some basic research on the organisations that you are going to approach before you make your application. It is rather pointless writing to a trust which only supports homeless people if your proposed project has nothing to do with providing accommodation. Similarly, it is a waste of time and effort to write for a donation of £2,000 if the trust you are approaching makes maximum grants of only £500. Publications like *The Directory of Grant-Making Trusts* will give you clear and accurate information about a whole range of grant-makers and will tell you what sort of projects they support, who to write to and how much they are likely to give.

In presenting your case, you will need to prepare written

information stating how essential your project is, why you need the money and what you will do with it when you get it. You will also need to demonstrate your capabilities as a group to carry out the things that you want to do. Your application, or appeal letter, is in fact an advertisement or promotion, which is designed to 'sell' your ideas to prospective donors. Make certain, then, that the following are evident in any bid that you make to seek out funding.

TELL THEM WHO YOU ARE

Use well-printed letter-headed paper to show that you are organised and have good standards of presentation. It is sometimes useful to have prominent and respected people as patrons whose names can be included on your written material. These can lend a degree of credibility to your group if you are fairly unknown. Make sure, however, that those whom you invite show that your organisation is well balanced in political, racial and gender terms. If, for example, you have decided to approach a Member of Parliament, then ensure that you have an MP from each political party. Essentially charitable trusts are not about politics or campaigns and you will do well to avoid seeking funds on the basis that you are a pressure group.

List the officers of your organisation and include a few lines on each of them about their backgrounds, and point out particularly any relevant experience or qualifications (not necessarily academic or professional) they may have for the task that you are embarking upon. Potential donors will need to be convinced that your group is:

a Honest.
b Able to see the job through to a successful conclusion.
c Able to spend any grant made economically and efficiently, giving value for money.
d Has access to any necessary expertise.

State that you are a registered charity (if indeed you are) and quote your charity number. State, too, in just a few sentences, the aims and objectives of your group.

TELL THEM WHAT YOU WANT TO DO

In an introductory paragraph or two explain briefly what the problem is at present, as you see it, perhaps giving a succinct overview of current government legislation or recommendations and how your proposed intervention will eliminate the difficulties that exist. In your attitude throughout, be confident and demonstrate that you believe strongly in what you are doing or attempting to do. Show that what you are proposing is both innovative and well thought through. Incorporating an apt quotation from a famous and valued person can sometimes help you to impress your point. Include a brief but pertinent personal story of someone who needs or has needed the service or facility that you are proposing and explain how you could help.

SELL YOUR IDEA TO THEM

Your application will need to include all your selling points, so before you actually write your application, brainstorm between you all the things you think your potential donor will find attractive and make sure that you find ways of including them in your letter of appeal. Read as much as you can about the policies of the organisations to whom you are going to make an application. Find out what their particular hobby horse is and emphasise the areas of your project that correspond. Check and double-check your application for simple things like layout and spelling errors. These may not seem important to you or what you are trying to achieve, but they may be important to others, and if these others are people who can influence the decision regarding your grant, then paying attention to details like this is worth the effort. Your application does not have to be a great glossy affair, but it does have to be presented well enough to convey your ability to do the job and to instil confidence in you.

Your application for funding will be greatly enhanced if you can manage to develop a sound reputation as a group. One way of doing this is to keep a note of all the successful things that your group does, so that you can mention them in any future applications. Make sure that you publicise your achievements in the local and national newspapers, television and so on. Keep a collection of any press cuttings and video recordings that you generate. You can send newsletter-type updates to councillors, Members of Parliament, newspapers, magazines and anyone who might be interested in what your group is doing. Make it your business to respond to news events by writing a well-constructed letter or offering to give your opinion on local television. Some of these things may put the fear of God into you at the moment, but it is surprising how quickly you can adjust and even learn to enjoy it. Of course, if you really can't bring yourself to be so prominent, there is always a well-articulated person around who can easily be persuaded to act as your spokesperson, provided that you take the time to enable him or her to become well versed in the issues.

Journalists are always on the look-out for a different slant on a particular event that has captured the public's attention, so it may be quite advantageous for you to think of links and angles that you can apply from the perspective of your particular cause and how it has a bearing. The 'home alone' features that have been appearing in the news a lot recently might, for example, be a way of bringing attention to your organisation which may perhaps be concerned about the way some residential institutions for children who have learning disabilities are understaffed and consequently are leaving very young, unqualified and inexperienced people to supervise children who are disabled.

You may also find it useful to monitor what others are doing in your field of work, like Local Authorities, perhaps, and make comparisons showing that what you are doing is more appropriate and generally much better.

THE NEED FOR EVALUATION

Many prospective sponsors will be more than interested in how you, as a group, will go about evaluating whether you are in fact meeting your own objectives. If, for example, you are asking for money to develop a supported employment initiative for youngsters in your area who have learning disabilities, then your aims and objectives will need to state specifically how many jobs you are hoping to create within the next twelve months and give some broad details about how you intend to gauge your success in achieving your aim. Having a credible independent person or organisation to assess your project to ensure that it is accomplishing what you intend is ideal and will no doubt be viewed favourably by donors whom you are approaching for funds. However, if you have to pay for such an evaluation, then it can be quite expensive. You therefore either have to build this cost into your application, or you will have to give a rough outline of the measures you are proposing to take, to reassure yourselves that the people for whom your scheme is intended are getting what they need, in the way that you planned. Another way of doing this is to design your own simple questionnaire so that you can get regular feedback from people who use your service or facility. This will give you the opportunity to see the strengths and weaknesses of what you provide and to change things accordingly. It will also reassure your fund-providers that their money is being well spent.

BE CLEAR ABOUT WHAT YOU ARE ASKING FOR

Include well laid out and well thought out calculations in respect of your group's projected income and expenditure. If you have been unable to get a qualified accountant as your treasurer, it is worthwhile asking someone who is used to finances professionally to help you in determining what you think your costs are going to be and to lay them out in a way which will be familiar to your potential benefactor.

When you write to anyone for funding, ensure that you

are specific about what you are asking them for, whether it be a specific amount of cash or an item that you require. Sometimes it is a good idea to provide a 'shopping list' of things that you need, showing a range of different costs. This way your sponsor can select something which is within its budget. When looking for a particularly large amount of money, I have in the past been successful by asking an organisation to give its commitment to providing, say, the last £5,000. This way the sponsor can be certain that it will only be asked to subscribe to your ambitious programme once you have managed to accrue all the rest of the money. Of course, this means that you can start with the advantage of saying that you need to raise X amount but that you already have £5,000 towards it, which shows other sponsors that you are capable of generating income even before you have approached them. This will certainly instil confidence in your organisation and make your fund-raising task that much easier.

SOME GENERAL POINTS ABOUT WRITING FOR MONEY

Keep your application as short and as simple as possible. There is bound to be lots of information that you want to include, but you will do well to be selective as the person to whom you are writing may well be getting dozens of applications to read every day; so make your application direct and to the point. You also need to write in plain English, avoiding the use of unnecessarily complex words and jargon. Remember, once you have written your proposal, read it over from the receiver's point of view. Including photographs, diagrams and so on can be a useful way of making your point and, at the same time, it can add to your document's overall presentation.

Don't expect to hear back from your possible sponsors immediately; a reply (if indeed you get one at all) may be a long time in coming. Some organisations will at least send you an acknowledgement of your application, but many do not, since postage is so expensive these days and they prefer to give their money to deserving causes rather than to the Post Office. I once wrote one hundred letters to trusts asking for money for a project that we were planning for young people who have a learning disability. Over a period of around three months, 62 replied expressing their regrets that they could not help, 33 did not reply at all and five sent cheques, which between them amounted to £15,000.

PUTTING ON A PROMOTION

Of course, you don't necessarily have to write letters in order to get funds. One way that I have found successful in the past is to invite others to raise funds for you. In one organisation of which I was a member, we made certain that we invited our town's mayor to be our patron each year. After a few years it became almost a tradition that the new mayor, in taking up office, would also become the new patron of our group. Amongst other things, this meant that we had access from time to time to the Mayor's Parlour, which was an impressive place and carried with it a certain amount of prestige. People were pleased to be invited there. This gave us unlimited opportunities, and on one occasion we sent invitations to over 250 publicans who had premises in the town, to a cheese and wine party in the Mayor's Parlour one weekday afternoon. Our wine and cheese was donated and use of the parlour was free. We prepared a simple video-tape which lasted for no longer than five or ten minutes, showing our problem and what we could do about it if we had enough money. We explained that it was for people who lived in our town. Then, of course, came the punch line. We were not asking them to make any donations, but if each of them were to go back to their pubs and put on an evening of fancy dress or perhaps a quiz night, then it would not be difficult for us to get the money we needed. If each pub put on only one of these nights and raised £100, then we would be able to accrue £25,000. The landlords and landladies found this an attractive idea, since they would not only be helping us, but would also be helping themselves by selling more beer.

Raising money can be fun, but one thing must remain paramount in your mind whilst doing it, otherwise you run the risk of defeating your own objects. It is essential that you never link disability with any action that might be seen to demean the people whom you are trying to resource. Getting funded is often very necessary, but should ensure that the dignity of those for whom the funds are intended is always maintained.

The essence of parent groups

Funding is merely a means to an end, and whilst the substance of cash is sometimes required, it should never be considered the most important aspect of what your group is about. Parents' groups are designed to support one another and to create opportunities for each other's sons and daughters who have learning disabilities. They do not have to run schemes, raise money, or even become very organised. There is always the danger that a small but effective informal group can become obsessed with its own administration and procedures to such a degree that it ends up being just another petty bureaucracy that cannot see the wood for the trees. Like anything else in life, your group should be firstly about people and relationships; anything else is only there to enable you and to empower you.

10 Living a Full Life of Their Own

> 'Often the impossible turns out to be just that which has not been attempted.'
> Ultimas Noticias

What most of us want in our own lives is peace of mind, good health, a sense of security, a degree of consistency, close links with our family and our circle of friends, a feeling of belonging and enough income to get by on. We want to be valued and respected. We want to know that someone cares. We want the chance to live a full life.

If this is what we would wish for ourselves, then it will not be surprising to learn that this is what people who have learning disabilities also want for themselves. But if you have learning disabilities, the real problem is that so many other people want to assume responsibility in deciding what you should or should not be allowed to do. That's fine when you are a child, but it can become pretty irritating, to say the least, when you find yourself in your early thirties and your mother is still telling you to wrap up warm before you go out, whilst licking her handkerchief and using it to wipe your face. While you are wanting to live life in the fast lane, everyone else keeps sticking their oar in, telling you to slow down. Of course, nobody wants to stand by and watch vulnerable people become exploited or put themselves at serious risk, but our concern for the welfare of people who have a disability all too often leads us into situations where, without realising the consequences, we somehow finish up dictating the terms and laying down the law.

Yes, some people need to be protected, but no one needs to be overprotected. Yes, some people need to have help in making *some* choices. No one needs to have *all* their choices always made for them. When parents have a child with learning disabilities, they need help and advice from various professionals. They need access to resources and to be empowered by learning new skills. What often happens is that these same professionals tell parents exactly what they must do and what resources will be given to them, and instead of being empowered to deal with their own situation, they are expected to become dependent upon State services. This 'I know what's best for you' attitude is frequently passed on to parents who continue to apply it to their sons and daughters.

Whether we like it or not, taking risks is central to our lives. Minimising the risk for the people we love is one thing, but maximising our control over them in order to achieve it is quite another. If we are not careful, those who are supposed to be our servants can turn out to become our tyrannical masters. Watching our nearest taking risks can somehow turn into a crisis in our own minds, which screams out for us to take action, but this action often prevents our children from opening up opportunities for themselves.

Our conservative western outlook prevents us from looking at a crisis situation in the same way that the Chinese do. They have a single written symbol for the word 'crisis' (see Figure 16) which is in fact made up of two symbols, one of which stands for danger and the other for opportunity. With their balanced philosophy represented by Yin and Yang, the Chinese long ago recognised that a crisis has two aspects, not just one. Here, in our own culture, we tend to focus only upon the danger element when the word crisis is mentioned, and fail to appreciate the other aspect which is opportunity. In the very centre of danger there is always opportunity, and at the very core of opportunity there will always be risk or danger.

In order to seize your opportunities in life, you also have

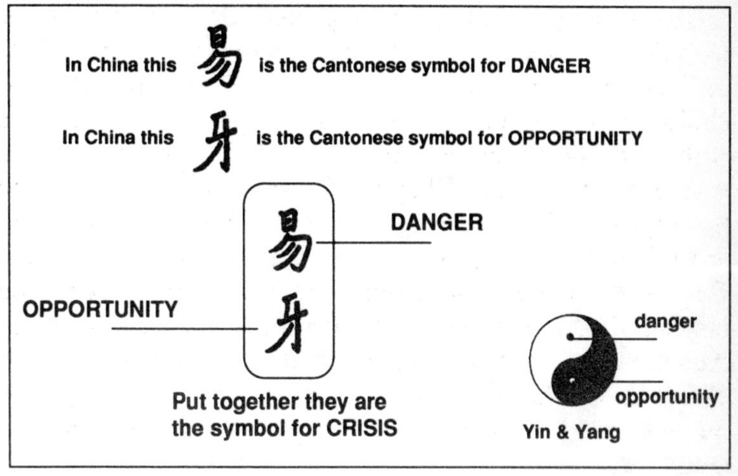

Figure 16. *Danger and opportunity.*

to tackle a degree of risk. If you decide that you will always avoid danger, then you will also be refusing to take opportunities that present themselves. The result will be a life which is narrow, limited and dull. In their attempts to keep their sons and daughters well insulated from the problems that the big ugly world outside can bring, many families unwittingly imprison young men and women in a lifestyle that leaves them severely restricted in all they do, and largely unfulfilled.

Both professionals and parents these days are struggling to shake off the old attitudes and restrictive practices which have in the past been the mainstay of the traditional institutions. Our fresh understanding of normalisation principles and the philosophy of INCLUSION is in line not only with central government thinking but, more to the point, with people's individual needs. We are beginning to learn about managing risk. In a service setting like a hospital or group home, this is usually erroneously interpreted as reducing the risk factors for managers and staff. They see themselves as the ones who get brought to book when things go wrong, so managing risk for them means keeping themselves well covered. Having a book of rules to go by, and sticking to them come what may, is one way to keep your career intact, but not often of much use to the person for whom you are supposed to be providing a service. Whilst it once seemed to fit in well with the old culture of institutionalisation, it no longer sits well with our more enlightened move towards the notion of INCLUSION and community belonging.

Today our risk management considerations must concern themselves with safeguarding the interests of the individual who has learning disabilities first and our own interests last. The Risk Indicator featured in Figure 17 shows that the more staff attempt to cut down on their own risk of being disciplined when things go wrong, or even could have gone wrong, the more they actually increase the risk of limiting the chances of the person for whom they are caring, to live a full and satisfying life. Times have changed, and our attitudes towards the way in which we support men and women who have learning disabilities have to change, too. Without risk there are no opportunities. Managing risk does not mean that we have to ensure that we eliminate risk altogether, it simply means that we should exercise our own judgement in calculating the amount of risk involved to the person for whom we have concern.

Even if we wanted, we could not do away with risk altogether. Everyone has times when they have to live a little dangerously; every day brings with it a fresh set of risks for all of us. According to the statistics, crossing the road is more hazardous than flying, but even just staying indoors is more dangerous than crossing the road or flying since most accidents happen in one's own home. Risks cannot be avoided, they are part and parcel of living on this planet. Whilst people who have learning disabilities will doubtless be more at risk than most, if we take it upon ourselves to see that they are always wrapped up in cotton wool, we only add to the difficulties they face in trying to live as full a life as possible. Not only will this mean a lifetime of worry and anxiety for ourselves in trying always to cover all the angles, but those whom we care for will only lose out.

RISK INDICATOR

DEGREE OF RISK	DEGREE OF RISK
For staff or parents getting blamed when things go wrong	For person who has learning difficulties having to live a completely unfulfilled life

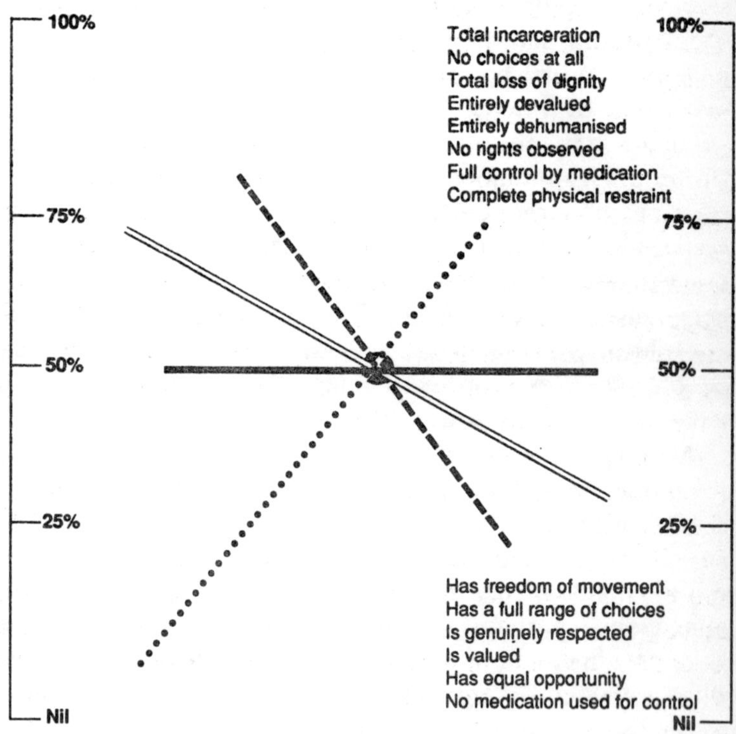

Figure 17. *The risk indicator.*

Using natural supports

We all need help in order to get by. Sometimes this comes in the form of various services, like social services and health services, but much of the time if comes from natural supports like friends and neighbours. For those who have a learning disability and have been placed firmly on the road to exclusion, special services are likely to be their only form of assistance, since they will not have had much opportunity to develop natural supports like friends and neighbours. In order to find natural support to surround an individual, a person must first be in his natural environment—that is to say, in his own home, in the community and preferably in a real job in the real world. The most under-utilised resource within our communities is people. People are abundant in their neighbourhoods and in all spaces and places. Extend invitations on behalf of your son or daughter. Let others know that he or she exists and has problems which, with their help, can easily be overcome. They will not know unless they are told. My own experience is that when you ask ordinary people to do extraordinary things they respond very well indeed. Be specific and be clear. A father may say:

'My son is now 18 years old and really enjoys going to the swimming pool, although he can't swim that well. Really he is too old to be going with his dad, but he doesn't have anyone else to go with.'

Tell friends who have sons the same age, approach swimming clubs—perhaps your local church will help. Be as creative as you can in letting as many people as possible know what is wanted. Eventually, in some way, somebody always responds. That person will recruit others and you will have to enable them by passing on all that you know about taking your son to the pool. You will probably have to accompany them to the pool on the first few occasions to satisfy yourself that they can cope and to give them the confidence to cope.

Of course, as a parent, it will not be easy for you to learn to let go. You are likely to feel that there is nobody else in the world who can look after your son as you can. You may also feel that it would be better to have a trained nurse around to make you feel a little easier. This is nonsense: nobody in the world needs medical assistance on hand twenty-four hours a day, unless he or she is in a coma. Remember, one day you will no longer be there, so other people have to learn to cope. You learned how; so can they.

People who have a learning disability need circles of friends more than anyone and they usually rely entirely upon you to initiate the introduction to some potential friends. Of course there are risks. There is no such thing as 100 per cent safety about anything, but developing a lifestyle based in the community involves no more risk than living in a separate institution. In fact, quite often, the dangers are less.

The natural support of friends and acquaintances who care can exist for your son or daughter if you allow it to. Effective support of this kind is not a technology that you can buy, or a professional service that is administered. It is something which is based upon values, people, relationships and circles. Natural support is about people who get involved, become committed, struggle and have fun together. Initiating a series of natural supports of this kind is one of the most effective things you can do to ensure that your son or daughter has the chance to live a full life.

The difference between service systems and community networks

Natural community networks of support are the much improved alternatives to the special services that are on offer. That is not to say that community networks can never be established with someone who has learning disabilities by service staff like social workers, or community nurses. They can, provided these professionals have a sound understanding of what is meant by real community networks. More often than not, professionals seem to think that community care is about starting a staffed scheme for a group of disabled people somewhere in the high street. This may be a way of starting, but it certainly isn't the be-all and end-all. What we are really aiming for is to ensure that individuals, not groups, are given every opportunity to participate fully in all that is going on in their own locality.

Institutions and various special service systems not only institutionalise those who use them, they institutionalise staff, too. Many professionals will tell you that they are developing their services on a model which is community based; however, in reality their own thinking has been influenced so much by the way they have provided services in the past that they are unable to understand fully the concept of community care or implement it without some form of bureaucratic control. Usually staff still see themselves as holding power and status rather than understanding that their role is one of enabling others and serving them. Steve Dowson, in his book *Moving to the Dance*, published by Values Into Action, listed a number of differences between a service culture and the way in which communities operate. This was based on the work of Bob Perske and John McKnight. Some examples are given below:

SERVICE SYSTEMS	COMMUNITY NETWORKS
Thrive on counting things and making reports.	Thrive on personal stories about real people.
Survive on money from above and are limited by budgets.	Will do some things with little or no money.
Humour tends to be ironic and displayed on notice-boards.	Laughter, celebrations and singing are from the heart.

Creativity can be controlled.	Creativity can be multiplied.
Usually take a distant view of tragedy and injustice.	Respond instantly by supporting victims of tragedy and injustice.
Thrive on assessing inabilities.	Thrive on recognising capabilities.
Orderly management is prized.	There is less order and people object to being managed.
Staff expect resources to be handed to them from above.	People work together with anything they have got.
Democracy is seen as impractical.	People value democracy.
Formality with standardised rules and roles is expected.	Informality with individualised face-to-face relationships is usual.
Services respond to designated priorities.	Local people respond quickly to one another.
Innovation is regarded with suspicion.	Creativity is normal and valued.
Often services require trained personnel to make them work. Anyone who falls short is seen as a barrier to a high quality service.	Ordinary people's talents are used optimally, without the expectation of perfection. All can play a part.

Leadership is usually ascribed to people in named positions.	Leadership functions are often shared amongst several people.
Perfection is sought with written plans and policies which often fail in their implementation because of human error. There is a reluctance for services to acknowledge their own errors, ignorance and fallibility.	People's imperfections are more readily acknowledged and people play to their strengths, aiming for the next step and at least minimising the worst that can happen.
Develop committees, task forces, advisory groups, multi-disciplinary teams, inspectorates, feasibility studies, assessment services and budget restrictions.	Real networks are small handfuls of people who mobilise on behalf of a person or family who is in trouble. The resources they use are little or no money, time, energy, telephones, comradeship, a strong determination to help, commitment and a fierce hunger for fair play.

In the past twenty years or so, professionals have had their goal posts changed. An ordinary life, as opposed to an institutionalised one, has been identified in various legislation as the new Holy Grail which has to be sought. Some professionals are adapting well, with a clear idea of where they are heading in terms of creating equal opportunity, greater choice and support to enable people who have learning disabilities to live their lives to the full. Others, however, remain stuck in the traditional special services mode and either refuse to make the change or fail to see how it can be done. Perhaps the worst are those who talk as if they support the view of developing an inclusive community, but in fact put all their efforts into providing the same things as they have always done.

Most Local Authorities have been focusing their attention upon changing places. They have been relocating people who have learning disabilities from hospital accommodation into ordinary houses and preparing them to use the same generic resources that we all share. Whilst they have learned a great deal about the mechanics of this process, they now need to explore further the infrastructure which exists in all communities, which will enable those who have additional needs to participate fully in local life and be included on an equal basis in their neighbourhood. It is this infrastructure that will determine to what degree a person becomes truly included. Just changing someone's address and placing him in his community is nowhere near enough; he also needs introductory help to establish his own circle of friends and day-to-day routines, and continued support to maintain them.

Parents, too, if they are not careful, can fall into the same trap as professionals, who often teach them that it is somehow safer or more advantageous to adopt a service attitude rather than follow their natural instincts to build community networks. Engage yourself and your son or daughter in all those things that lead towards an ordinary life based in the local neighbourhood, and avoid anything which separates you into something which is called special. Do the common-sense thing every time, rather than the bureaucratic thing. Make your own judgements about people; they will tell you far more than a police check. Don't rely upon a person's qualifications to impress you; a caring neighbour can often be far more reliable than a trained professional. Don't take senseless risks, but do take reasonable risks. If we are to make real progress in enriching the lives of those who have additional needs, whether as a parent or as a professional, we have to learn to free ourselves from thinking in traditional service ways and begin to discover more about the process of INCLUSION.

Traditionally we are used to:
situations where we have control and power over.
INCLUSION means that we:
need to learn more about collaboration and negotiation.

Traditionally we see people:
as needing to be fixed.
INCLUSION means that we:
must start to recognise people's strengths and gifts.

Traditionally we are used to:
staffing places and supervising people.
INCLUSION means that we:
have to learn how to facilitate the involvement of friends and neighbours.

Traditionally we are used to:
dictating the terms and rules.
INCLUSION means that we:
have to learn how to give those who have additional needs more choices and opportunities.

Traditionally we are used to:
devising programmes, implementing behaviour modification and other intrusive therapy.
INCLUSION means that we:
must learn the benefits of allowing people with learning disabilities to have normal experiences as opposed to abnormal ones.

Traditionally we are used to:
grouping people together according to their ability or behaviour.
INCLUSION means that we:
have to start to realise the benefits of diversity.

Traditionally we are used to:
seeing people as having bits missing or broken.
INCLUSION means that we:
need to see people as complete and whole just as they are.

Further education and higher education

My son Adam and my daughter Mandy could hardly wait to break out of school at the age of sixteen in order to start living their lives as adults. They both assumed that this would give them more recognition of their own maturity and a chance to earn money. This income, of course, along with their new-found status as wage earners, would, they calculated, enable them to have a degree of independence not previously within their grasp.

By the age of nineteen, both of them had kept their eyes on the main chance and taken the plunge by getting themselves careers, a long-term relationship with a partner of their own age and a hefty mortgage on a modest dwelling. Not everybody's idea of fun, perhaps, but it was certainly what they wanted and now, three years later, they would readily tell you that they have learned more about the practicalities of life and surviving than they would ever have gained from attending any education course. By the age of sixteen they were sick of chalk and talk, and so headed for citizenship rather than studentship.

It is a personal choice, of course, and for a plethora of reasons many choose to go on into further or higher education. There is no right or wrong answer, just choice and personal preference. Youngsters who have learning disabilities have this same choice, but for most of them further education means another two or three years at college with the same disabled people with whom they have already spent most of their lives. On the whole, further education for many people is seen as a second chance. It's a place where you go to have another stab at your exams or to learn the things that you didn't quite grasp the first time round. It is, however, quite different from school, in that it has a more adult environment—unlike sixth form colleges which, try as they may, have strong roots in school. Youngsters go into further education either on a vocational or a non-vocational basis, vocational meaning that they are aiming for particular career or job opportunities, as opposed to non-vocational where they can follow their own particular interests.

The 1988 Education Act has made it clear to colleges that they should have regard for people who have learning disabilities, but like everything else this has become a matter of interpretation. Whilst some establishments are taking steps to access the same course for all students, others are happy to say that the needs of people who have learning disabilities are being met in the further education departments of special schools. All colleges, however, now have to have a policy statement and a named person at the college who has a particular responsibility to answer questions about what they provide for those who have additional needs.

Since the 1991 Education Act, colleges have become independent and now rely upon their funding from the Further Education Funding Council (FEFC). This body expects them to have a clear understanding of their students' destinations. Colleges now need to have definite goals for their students and must not merely be interested in recruiting numbers as they were in the past. The Further Education Funding Council has a policy steer towards INCLUSION and one hopes only fully fund those establishments which have true destinations for their students and are giving those who have additional needs access to the same courses, fundamentally, like everyone else. Currently there are already around 100,000 students who have learning disabilities using further education facilities.

Higher education refers to the universities which offer degree courses. For most of these, the glittering prizes are reserved only for those capable of high academic achievement, and the words 'university' and 'learning difficulty' are quite incompatible. Nevertheless, Bolton Institute of Higher

Education is leading the way when it comes to including students who have learning disabilities. Like many other academic establishments, its degree courses are modular and continuous assessment has replaced examinations. Bolton Institute is about to offer a Master of Arts degree in 'Educational Issues Around Learning Disability', with modules like 'Sexuality and Learning Disabilities'. There is an access officer and student services at Bolton, which will help those who have learning disabilities to participate in any of the modules available. They do not have to complete the whole degree course. Joe Whittaker, who is a senior lecturer and the main force behind implementing these exciting opportunities, says that having people who themselves have learning difficulties enrolling on the course will be a tremendous advantage for everyone. Each module lasts around fifteen weeks and costs around £50. Joe Whittaker can foresee a time when practical non-academic degrees will be made available in universities and other higher education establishments.

Real jobs

One of the factors that establishes us as a person in our own right is having a proper job. By that I mean one that actually needs to be done, as opposed to one which is artificially created simply to keep someone occupied. Apart from enabling you to earn money, a real job can give you satisfaction, a chance to be valued for what you do and opportunities to extend your network of friends, acquaintances and contacts. Many people meet their future husbands and wives at work.

For those who have learning disabilities, the options after leaving school or further education can often be extremely limiting. They tend to get caught between the ignorance and prejudice of prospective employers and the low expectations held about them by staff in the special services that are designed to help them. Adult training centres are usually the places they are expected to attend. These represent a path to further exclusion which is often determined for them long before they leave school. Once again, these are facilities which cater only for people who have disabilities and so restrict their chances of fully interfacing with the rest of us in their own communities.

Adult training centres are run by Social Services and are staffed by people called instructors. For years they have been called training centres, but the odd thing is that nobody ever seemed quite sure what the nature of the training was. It certainly didn't equip people for real jobs, since very few who attended a training centre ever left it. This in itself created problems for some Local Authorities, who found that as ten or twenty youngsters left their special schools each year, the adult training centre, built for a hundred 'trainees', was fast becoming oversubscribed since nobody ever moved on at the other end. The more myopic Local Authorities began to build on extensions, only to find that a further extension was needed just a year or two later.

Nowadays there is a greater understanding of the need to enable those who have a learning disability to become skilled in areas which enable them to seek open employment with a degree of confidence. Some forward-thinking organisations have been exploring the alternatives to adult training centres and have invested time, money and effort in supported employment, with a great deal of success. This concept began in America more than ten years ago and because of it over 100,000 people who have learning disabilities now hold down real jobs. Companies like Boeing now actually employ full-time supported employment consultants, and Pizza Hut insist that all their outlets in the State of California take on at least one person through a supported employment scheme. Unlike the idea behind adult training centres, supported employment does away with the notion of 'preparing readiness for work', for we have seen that readiness in this sense rarely seems to come for the person who has learning disabilities, but will invariably keep the instructors well employed until pensionable age. Supported employment also does away with the idea of 'prevocational training' and 'work experience'. Effectively people are now recognising that anyone can work productively, provided he or she has enough of the relevant help that she needs to learn and maintain her function as an employee.

The idea of supported employment, therefore, is to help people who have additional needs to acquire and maintain a real job which they enjoy, paid at a fair rate and based in the regular work place. Supported employment cuts out the unnecessary middle man, which in this case happens to be adult training centres. There is no virtue in spending years in training without ever getting a job at the end of it. Supported employment allows people who have learning disabilities to be trained on the spot to do work which they like and for which they are paid.

STATUS EMPLOYMENT

This organisation is based in Croydon, Surrey. Kimberley Charman and Tony Coggins are the driving force which put it together. They find real jobs for people who have learning disabilities and then send one of their consultants on site to learn precisely what is involved in doing that job. Once they have grasped what is required, they proceed to teach the employee at the work place for however long it takes him or her to learn—a day, a week, a month or longer. The consultant also ensures that the employee will pick up all the day-to-day routines at work and the culture of the place, so that he will find it easier to slot himself in. The consultant remains in regular contact with both the employer and employee, so that he or she is always on hand to help with any unforeseen difficulties which might arise.

The benefits to the employee are obvious, but there are also considerable advantages for the employer. The systematic training approach that is used provides the employer with personnel who have the necessary skills, together with other assets like complete reliability, attention to detail and loyalty. These are qualities which make it an attractive proposition for companies to meet their legal obligations to include in their work force people who have disabilities.

John is one of the many people who have used supported employment to get themselves a real job. John is 29 years old and, like many other people who have learning disabilities, attended an adult training centre on a full-time basis from the time he left school. He did the usual things there like packing things into boxes, doing some art and craft work and playing various sports. Whilst he enjoyed sport, twelve years of it is enough for most people, and after a while John was seen as disruptive and certainly unemployable. At home he had caring parents who had got into the routine of making all his decisions for him. They chose the clothes he wore, told him where and when he was to go on holiday and vetted his friends, approving some but not others. The rest of John's life was controlled by other people who were paid to look after him.

In just three weeks John was trained to carry out a real job in a department store; but more than that, he learned how to use public transport, which gave him the opportunity to move around from A to B without having to wait for someone to take him. He discovered a new circle of friends with whom he now spends his leisure time, and for the first time in his life he brought home a pay packet. He took his parents out for a meal and was quite definite that in future he wanted to wear jeans. Now he thinks that, with some support, he will be able to do what most other youngsters do—move into his own place.

Rebecca was the first person to contact Status Employment to find her real employment. At the age of 22 years she was coming to the end of her college course for people who have special needs. The fact that she had been born with Down's syndrome meant that she had been directed towards segregated services for most of her life. Her mother had always tried her best to involve her daughter in real life, but this had not been easy due to the separations that she had been placed in by the special system. Now she had come to the end of all this special education, and where had it left her? With few relevant skills and not much prospect of a glittering future.

Kimberley Charman became Rebecca's employment consultant and began by putting together a personal vocational profile. This was a way of bringing together all the relevant information that would help them to choose the best job match. Kimberley got to know more about Rebecca by meeting her several times, sometimes alone, sometimes with her family present, sometimes with her friends, and visited her when she was carrying out some voluntary work, ironing clothes in a charity shop. These were all ways of gleaning valuable information. Just any old paid employment was not good enough: Rebecca was looking for some part-time shop work in the Croydon area, where she could meet other people of her own age.

Between them they established that Rebecca liked fashionable clothes and make-up and that she enjoyed dance, aerobics and styling her hair. Kimberley was able to arrange for her to spend some time on the shop floor at Marks & Spencers just before Christmas, as a sales assistant in their gifts and toiletries department. There were no vacancies for a permanent post, but they decided that at least she would be able to see if this was the kind of job she would like. Rebecca thoroughly enjoyed it all, and when she turned up for the second time, the management offered her a permanent job in gifts and toiletries for two days each week, starting in January.

CO-OPTIONS LTD. COMMUNITY CO-OPERATIVE

Co-options began around four years ago in North Wales, in an area of extremely high unemployment, which rates among the top two per cent of the most deprived areas in the United Kingdom. They set themselves the task of forging strong links between people who have learning disabilities and the business world, with four major considerations uppermost in their minds:

1 Vision. Thinking about desirable futures with individuals.
2 Identifying an individual's gifts, interests and needs.
3 Developing appropriate supports and safeguards.
4 Making new connections in the community.

They went about achieving these aims by using the company to launch a number of small enterprises. Whilst each of these had to make a profit in order to survive, their main aim was to create inclusive community-based work opportunities for local people who have learning or multiple disabilities and who in the past have only ever been offered places like special care units in which to spend the rest of their lives. Since 1989, Co-options has grown steadily and has now created eight new businesses:

1 Tangible Dream, a business covering mountain bike repair, retail, hire and outdoor adventures.
2 Café Ciao Bella, a quality whole food café and outside catering business.
3 Co-options Supported Employment Services, a registered employment agency which now employs over 20 job coaches. This company works closely with Social Services and other agencies to develop supported employment opportunities.
4 Magic Toy Box Nursery, Denbigh.
5 Magic Toy Box Nursery, St Asaph.
6 Magic Toy Box Nursery, Rhyl.
   These three companies are work place nurseries. Co-options now operates its own low-cost franchises.
7 Mosaic, an art studio which has facilities like a darkroom, silk screen printing equipment and a comfortable environment in which to work and relax.
8 Essentially Celtic markets a range of aromatherapy oils and associated products like books, candles and burners. There is a part-time aromatherapist on site, who is available for consultation. Currently Essentially Celtic

employs ten people, three of whom have learning disabilities.

Two of the above companies have now been launched independently and operate in their own right outside the original umbrella organisation of Co-options Ltd. Nevertheless, they are charged to remain firmly committed to the initial goals.

Co-options Ltd. now has business partners all over Europe and the United Kingdom, including Eire, Portugal, Germany and Greece, and are still expanding. The company also offers a consultancy service to other people who would like to start up a supported employment organisation like theirs. They have a fund-raiser who can develop bids with organisations on a contingency fee basis, and they run a number of training courses in small business development, framework for accomplishments, training in supported employment, as well as more specialised business planning in project design and development. Their address can be found at the end of this book.

Housing

Everyone needs somewhere to live, and for most families this means that their children will grow into young adults, become fledgelings and fly the nest in order to make a nest of their own, and perhaps make a family of their own, too. Some simply feel it is time to have their own pad and leave the household to form a coalition with some of their friends so that they can rent an 'economical' place together, the like of which their parents tremble at, and when they see their chosen décor they very often tremble even more. Others leave home when they become full-time students and live in halls of residence. Whatever way it is done, most youngsters seem to leave the old homestead, somewhere between their late teens and mid-twenties.

Many parents of youngsters who have learning disabilities, however, tend to hang on to their children, rather as a tug of war team hangs onto the rope. The outcome can only be detrimental for parents and offspring. As the parents get older, they also become less able to cope with all the day-to-day responsibilities that they impose upon themselves. They tend to tire more easily, and their son or daughter grows more resentful at being continually treated as a child, with no real life of his or her own. The outcome is invariably much the same. Parents eventually die, and those whom they leave behind are consigned to the Local Authority's residential accommodation. No one is happy.

Buying or renting their own home is not out of the question simply because people have additional needs. What it requires is a good circle of friends, some creative thinking and the will of parents to let your youngsters grow up and take a well-supported step in the direction of independent living. One thing you can do, which costs absolutely nothing, is to get your son's or daughter's name on the council's housing list as soon as possible. In most places there is a long waiting list of some years, so why not get your child's name down as soon as he or she is sixteen? It's amazing just how many people never consider doing this—they seem to think that their children's disability somehow precludes them.

Some people worry that a house might actually become available—what then? Well, get the offer of a house first and you can work out how your son or daughter will be supported thereafter. Once a house is on the cards, it is astounding how this can focus your attention and get you thinking creatively. If your son or daughter is unemployed and on a low income, he or she will qualify for housing benefit from the local council and you may find that you can work out a viable way of using this benefit, along with other people's (not necessarily people who have learning disabilities) in order to give your son or daughter a chance of living independently from you. This can be done in collaboration with a housing association, perhaps, or with a private property owner.

Your son's or daughter's claim for housing benefit is assessed by a council employee who makes a judgement on what he considers a fair rent for the property that your child is proposing to occupy. In fact 95 per cent of this is paid by central government and the remaining five per cent by the local council. There are situations in which housing benefit can be topped up, with half being met by central government and the other half by the local council, so don't be put off by properties which you think might be too expensive to rent. If the local council cannot find anywhere for your son or daughter to rent at the proposed benefit rate, which completely meets his or her additional needs, then the law insists that a top-up must be made.

Leisure

Much of the quality of a person's life is determined by the way he uses his spare time. Generally speaking, most of us spend about a third of our day sleeping, a third working and the remaining third at leisure. Leisure is the global term we use to refer to the total period of time that we spend relaxing—Chambers' *Twentieth Century Dictionary* describes it as 'time free from employment and occupation'. How we spend it varies considerably for each of us: from very passive and informal pastimes like sipping coffee with friends, through to the more energetic extreme of organised sports such as squash rackets or aerobics.

Few of us would want to spend the whole of the leisure third of our day entirely in organised active recreation, any more than we would relish devoting it all to reclining in an armchair watching television or reading the newspaper, without feeling the need to get up and do something a bit more taxing. We therefore, whether consciously or not, tend to balance our allocation of leisure time with a mix of organised and informal events, active and inactive, whichever suits our mood and personal choice. Having someone round to watch the big match on television with you, or being invited to a friend's house for a cup of tea, are leisure time activities which can hold at least as much social significance as joining the local swimming club or football team.

The leisure preferences of people who have learning disabilities are no different; nevertheless, for many of them there are always those people around who are trying to organise them by ensuring that they have something active to occupy their minds. On the other hand, they may find that they are left for hours on end in their rooms, away from everyone else, to watch television. Of course people need time to themselves and, from choice, some of our leisure time is spent on our own, simply relaxing and doing nothing in particular. But people who have learning disabilities also need the opportunity to develop new interests, meet different people and share their interests with others of the same age.

Leisure time activities are a good way of making new friends, but too often, with those who have additional needs, the interest or activity is regarded by others as an end in itself and the importance of the opportunity to develop other relationships is not fully considered. This becomes particularly apparent when your son or daughter is found 'volunteers' to take him or her swimming, horse riding or whatever. On the whole, volunteers are quite different from friends and neighbours: the person next door who helps out by bringing you a cooked meal when you are temporarily incapacitated is viewed quite differently from the meals-on-wheels brigade who, on the face of it, do exactly the same job. Valuable as they are and caring as they can be, the very fact that they have volunteered to enable you to indulge your hobby or interest makes a statement about you as an object of charity, rather than someone who has friends with whom you share your leisure time.

When you have a learning disability, the notion of a volunteer carries with it a stigma, a suggestion of unequal relationships and, possibly, patronising attitudes. There are times, of course, when compromises have to be made and using a volunteer may be the only way to get your son or daughter to the local youth club, aerobics course or whatever. However, you need to remember that volunteers should only be a temporary means to an end: the real aim is to have your son or daughter fully included in the club and that, given time, others will be encouraged to consider and deal with the additional needs which have to be met in ensuring that their new member participates like everyone else.

If you need a volunteer at all, he or she should be employed in the role of facilitator—someone who not only takes your son to wherever he needs to go, but introduces him to other people, develops his confidence and instils in him a sense of belonging; who helps him overcome some of the simple, everyday difficulties that he has to deal with in order to be there and participate. A good facilitator gently and subtly encourages others jointly to understand, accept and meet the needs of their new colleague. A good facilitator also knows when to keep a low profile. By remaining beside the disabled person the whole time, he or she can act as a barrier and inhibit the natural inclination of others to stop and talk or offer their assistance. A constant companion in evidence may lead other people to assume that everything the disabled person needs will be dealt with, and so they never seek to take on any helping role themselves.

Settling down—getting married

Marriage is an institution, they say, but who wants to live in an institution? The fact is, fewer people are getting married these days and of those who do the divorce rate is remarkably high—something like one in three. Whatever our preference, we now seem to have a greater number of choices when it comes to the way we conduct our permanent personal relationships, all of which, by and large, appear to be quite socially acceptable. We can live together for a while before getting married, in order to 'test it out', or we can just live together without feeling the need to get married at all. Children born out of wedlock no longer carry a stigma, and having once sent people to prison for homosexuality, we are now learning to accept that gay people have a right to live together and even adopt children. Of course, there are still a few old romantics left like Sheila and myself, who put themselves through the marriage ceremony (photographs, confetti and all), but we put that down to our conditioning rather than anything else. The point is, if these are the choices available to couples nowadays, why would we want to prevent people who have an intelligence quotient that is lower down the scale than the rest of us, from having the same choices? The fact is, you wouldn't believe the horror that some people express at the thought of those who are considered to be 'mentally handicapped' getting married or living together.

'But what if sex rears its ugly head?' they say, or:

'Oh God, what if they have children?'

Of course people who have learning disabilities can and do settle down together, get married sometimes and have their own family. As far as I am aware, we don't have a law that prevents people from doing this just because their IQ score is less than our society thinks it ought to be—though, quite amazingly, the 1983 Mental Health Act does make it illegal for *anyone* to have sex with someone who is offensively referred to as 'defective' (see page 179). On the other hand, perhaps there should be a law to prevent others from interfering in their personal lives and continually narrowing their options. If we consider that only able-bodied people, or those who have an average or above average intellectual ability, can be good spouses or parents, I can show you plenty of evidence that would dispel this theory. Break-ups and divorce among 'ordinary folk', as well as child abuse and neglect, are sadly far too commonplace for us to claim that a certain amount of intelligence is required in order to express our love and caring.

Recently I spoke to Les and Mary who have both been labelled as having learning disabilities. They met each other back in November 1975 when Les was just 29 years old and Mary was 20. A few years after his mother died, Les found that living alone with his father was not working out as well as he had hoped, and after approaching the Social Services in his locality, he was given residential accommodation along with 31 other people who also had learning disabilities. One of these residents was Mary. By October 1981 Les and Mary had started spending time together. They would go to their local pub at least once a week and often went to places like the cinema and theatre together. In 1984 Les moved to a group home which he shared with Jack and Ronald. He still saw a great deal of Mary who spent most evenings with him.

Les and Mary knew each other for four years before Les popped the question. Expressing their wish to get engaged meant that a meeting had to be held with staff where they were living and with Mary's mother. By this time, Les's father had died. People at this meeting recognised and acknowledged just how much Mary and Les cared for each other and the engagement went ahead. This was December 1985 and Les was now 39 and Mary 30. Mary's mother went to a number of jewellers with Les and her daughter, looking at engagement rings, pointing out the ones she liked. Later in the day, Les took Mary and his future mother-in-law for a pub lunch and, during the meal, produced a small box which he placed on the table and opened. It contained a sparkling engagement ring that Mary and Les had bought together some days before. Mary's mother laughed and called them both 'crafty devils'.

Although they had got engaged, there was no date set for a wedding. Like so many people these days, they moved into a flat and lived together for the following six years. However, in 1992 they got married in their local registry office and spent their honeymoon at the seaside. When they celebrated their first wedding anniversary they were asked if they had ever thought about divorce. They both smiled, hugged each other and said in a most definite way, 'No way!'

11 Good Grief—Don't Run Away from It

'Blessed is the person who is too busy to worry in the daytime and too sleepy to worry at night.' Leo Aikman

Paradoxically, whilst life itself is always uncertain, there is nothing more sure than death. Whoever we are, death is inevitable. It's a sobering thought that, as soon as we are born, we begin to die. No one lives forever and yet few of us seem at all well prepared for the grand final event when it comes, either for ourselves or for those whom we love. Somehow death nearly always catches us out and happens when we least expect it. And when it does, there is always somebody somewhere who will be heard to say, 'Well, you never know what's round the corner, do you?' And yet of course we *do* know exactly what's round the corner, but we choose to ignore it. It's rather like the fact that we always seem to get snowed up during winter in the UK. Snow ploughs are never at hand when they are most needed. When interviewed on television, after a day of total chaos on the roads, some civil servant from the Highways and Byways Department will look shocked and say, 'Snow in January! Well, who would have thought it?'

Personally, I never really gave much consideration to death at all, until my father died. Like everyone else, I was too busy getting on with the day-to-day trivia that I made so artificially important. Then a bolt came from the blue one day, when I received a call to say that Dad had sustained a cardiac arrest from which, I later discovered, he had not recovered. It was difficult to comprehend—after all, I had been with him just the day before and he had seemed as fit as a butcher's dog. So it was hard to take in. Death had never really been amongst the words that we had used with each other. I didn't know what he thought about death and the after-life, or even that for years he had carried with him a kidney donor card. Dying is not something that people discuss a lot. We had never talked about whether he had a preference for burial or cremation, or any of the hundred and one other things that surround the end of your life. Somehow, death had become a taboo subject, something that was regarded as 'not nice' to talk about, like group sex or bodily functions. But it is an unnecessary taboo that needs to be overcome.

The passing away of someone close to you establishes in your own mind a much clearer concept of your own mortality. Undoubtedly it sharpens the focus on your personal life and puts things in a more meaningful perspective. For a while at least, somebody else's death can help you to readjust your own values and develop a more profound set of priorities. If you are a workaholic, for instance, it may make you realise that no one on their death bed ever said, 'I wish I had spent more time at the office'! As far as we know, we have only one life and, like it or not, this is it. If the Bible is anything to go by, then we can reasonably expect to have at our disposal some three score years and ten. Well, it is happening to you right now. This is not a dress rehearsal, this is life and the clock has already started.

Grieving is as much part of our emotional repertoire as laughing and happiness. It is a process which is necessary for us to go through when someone close to us is no longer around any more. Whether we grieve for the person who has gone, or for ourselves because our own life is perceived as being worse off without that person, I am uncertain. Nevertheless, grief certainly has a role to play in helping us make the necessary adjustment, so that we can continue with the rest of our own life.

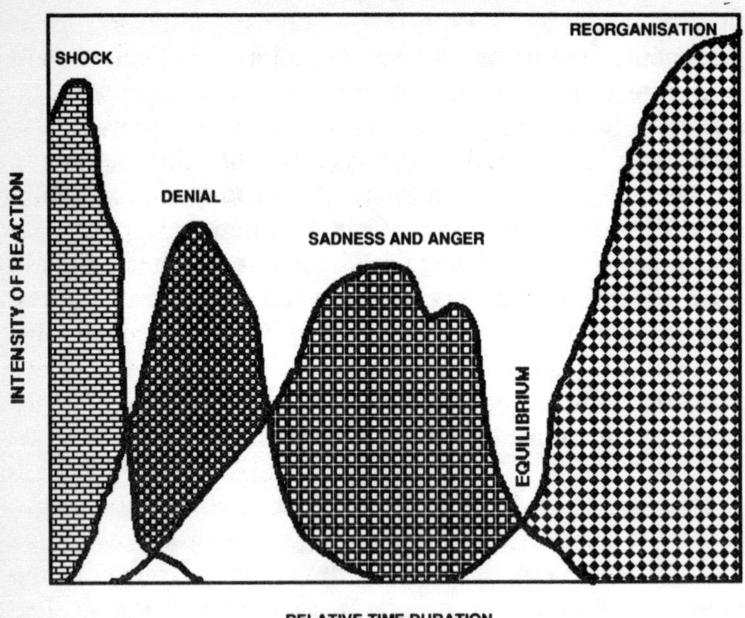

Figure 18. *The grieving process.*

The diagram shown in Figure 18 is the same one that was used in Figure 4 (see p. 26). This is no accident. It simply underlines the fact that the outline process of grief is much the same, whether it is applied to mourning the loss of someone close to you through death, or whether it is from the loss of the 'perfect' baby to whom you expected to give birth. In trying to gain some idea of what a person with learning disabilities (or anyone else, for that matter) will be going through, this same grief model will give some overall guidance about the general process people experience when a serious loss occurs in their lives. Each of these stages will be felt in different intensity by different people, and individuals will vary considerably in the amount of time they spend going through them.

SHOCK

Shock can be a useful defence mechanism, which acts as a buffer for events that may be extremely traumatic. It gradually lets in the reality, at a pace which allows the person to cope, both emotionally and physically. Just like the rest of us, people who have considerable intellectual limitations experience the effects of shock. Often their suffering is not recognised or appreciated, even by those who know them well. Sometimes their need to mourn is either not even considered or is dismissed as being completely unnecessary due to their disability. Denying people the opportunity to grieve for their loss can not only have serious consequences for them, but is an act of emotional brutality.

Being off their food, showing weight loss, withdrawal and bizarre behaviours are some of the more obvious signs of emotional upheaval, but there are many others for which you need to be on the look-out. These are likely to be specific to the people themselves, signs which only their friends, family and others close to them will notice—failing to take an interest in things which they usually enjoy, for instance, or perhaps not responding to personal routines in the way they usually do. For some people, reaction to shock may take an acute physical form: they may vomit, feel faint, shake, become breathless, have a choking sensation or become cold and shivery. Physical symptoms of this kind may be particularly severe when the death has been sudden and totally unexpected or when the griever has actually witnessed it. Recalling in the mind's eye aspects of the death, such as the look on the person's face or the thought that he or she might have suffered badly, is likely to prolong this stage of shock and be extremely upsetting for the one left to mourn. Numbness is a feature which many people describe at a time like this, and a feeling of unreality. For many, it seems that whilst they are aware of all that is going on around them, they feel that they are somehow not part of it, but are just looking down on what is taking place, like some out of the body experience. It is as though they are on automatic pilot.

Signs of shock in those who have great difficulty in communicating their thoughts and feelings particularly need to be watched for at times of loss. They need the comfort and reassurance of a cuddle and physical closeness as much as anyone else, if not more. What they don't need is to be formally referred to some professional who thinks that a behaviour modification programme will be the answer. No programmes or treatments, just sensitivity and some genuine understanding, are usually what is called for. Where grief is concerned, responding as a caring human being is the most useful thing that anyone can do. Shock for most people is overcome relatively quickly and often does not last much past the funeral.

DENIAL

After shock there may well come a period of disbelief. Your daughter may seek out the person who has died in all the usual places where he used to be. She may still lay a place for him at table, or try to visit him or call him on the phone. These are times when you can only be honest and reiterate that the person for whom she is looking has died and won't be returning. Be truthful about this, no matter how much your daughter may shout her denials to you. It is a good idea to try to get her to express her grief in some tangible way, like laying flowers on the grave or writing a letter. Ritual is important and so engaging in all the traditional routines surrounding death is essential. That is why it is advisable for you to refrain from excluding someone who has learning difficulties from attending the funeral, eating the ham sandwiches, revisiting the grave and so on, so that she has had the same opportunities as you to participate in all the practical elements of laying the deceased to rest. The false idea that you are in some way protecting your daughter by keeping her away from sad occasions will only help to exacerbate denial. Being up-front about things, and including people with learning difficulties in all of the procedures, will give them a chance to understand and, in time, adapt.

SADNESS AND ANGER

Inner emotional pain is intense, often causing insomnia, uncontrollable sobbing and total restlessness. People who have learning disabilities need a great deal of support at this time, but unfortunately they often simply do not get it. Once the immediate shock has been overcome and the practicalities of the funeral completed, friends tend to feel that the state of mourning is largely over. Those grieving may feel that they should no longer display their feelings publicly, and confine their sadness to times when they are alone. Our Western culture seems to deter us from airing our emotions for too long, and men in particular may feel that tears should only be shed privately, when they are on their own.

Whilst some mourners need to spend moments by themselves, leaving them alone for too long is not advisable. The person who is grieving may well benefit from having something concrete to hang on to, such as making a scrapbook of memories or having a photo of the deceased enlarged and framed to keep in his or her bedroom. Talk about the dead person, too, recalling some of the good and bad times that were shared; recognise his existence and some of the things for which he was known.

Those in grief may quite irrationally blame the death of the deceased on somebody in particular. They may feel guilt because they see themselves as having somehow played a part, or they may point the finger at the attending doctor or perhaps even yourself. Anger will be expressed at whoever they hold responsible and often the person grieving becomes in danger of falling out with those whom they need most, but if you can see this through with some patience and understanding, then this phase will pass. Similarly, they may feel deserted by the person who has died and aim their frustrations against him. Feelings are better expressed than repressed, so do let people who are grieving be aware that it is all right to be angry, irritable or to cry, if that is what they want to do. Do your best to ensure that they get every opportunity to continue with the same routines as always.

If, for instance, they normally go to a club on Wednesday evenings and still feel like going, then don't stand in their way. They will need the security of familiar things, so making changes in their life at this time is usually not helpful.

EQUILIBRIUM

If people have been supported by the openness and honesty of those around them, have managed to keep all the other aspects of their life continuing in much the same way as always, like going to the same places and meeting the same people as they normally do, then eventually they will be able to gather themselves together and deal with their inner turmoil in a more practical way. They will begin to pick up the pieces and, bit by bit, start to carry on with their lives.

REORGANISATION

Finally, in their own time and way, they will reach the stage of reorganisation where they have learned to accept the situation and are carrying on their day-to-day activities without being under stress or duress. Of course, this is not the complete end to the story. Recovering from grief can be just as difficult as all the other stages. It is a time when the griever has to pull back on some of the emotional energy which he or she has used in the past and begin to invest it in new relationships for the future. This is not as easy as it might sound since the making of new relationships involves some risk. There is a danger of rejection, for one thing, or the act of making fresh companions could generate feelings of disloyalty to the deceased. When people have recently experienced bereavement, they are emotionally very vulnerable and easily susceptible to being hurt again. Most people learn to adjust, but almost everyone will feel the pain of the earlier stages from time to time. Something may trigger it off, like an anniversary or birthday, perhaps. Nevertheless, they will have discovered how to cope and these feelings of melancholy that come upon them from time to time, with insight and support from others, are likely to be fairly short-lived. Life goes on!

* * *

This process of mourning that I have outlined is merely an overall guide to give you a general framework of understanding about how all people deal with their feelings of loss. Reactions and behaviour will be significantly different from person to person, whether they have a disability or not. When we grieve we all feel sorrow, but we feel it and express it in different ways. Not only does the speed of true realisation that a loved one has died vary considerably from one individual to another, but the intensity of our anguish will be felt in different ways and at different levels. Added to that, our response to a loss will take a range of forms. Whilst some of us will weep bitterly on and off for a considerable length of time, others will become angry or perhaps very quiet and withdrawn. Some will want to busy themselves doing just about anything, whilst others will collapse in a chair and simply go into themselves.

There is no right response at a time like this. Those who are in mourning do not have to behave in the way that you behaved or that you think they should behave. Coping with loss is done in our own way and we cannot change that. Rather like the individuality of fingerprints, we each have our own way of dealing with our losses. It is no good trying to get people to cry just because you think that it is the healthy thing to do, or try to force them out of themselves. Grieving will take as long as it takes and will find its own way of coping. Have no illusions about it, people who have learning difficulties, no matter how severe and no matter what age, are no different when it comes to feeling grief and loss. There are however, a number of things that you can take into consideration when helping someone through this difficult time.

Always be honest about it

Some people have the quaint idea that they have a role in life to protect their disabled son or daughter from all the pain in the world. This misconception is doomed to fail for just about everyone concerned. Trying to take on all the heartache for somebody else leads only to constant over-anxiety for yourself and at the same time prevents your youngster from learning about his or her existence and finding out how to cope with it in the same way that everyone else has to. Particularly when it comes to the subject of the death of somebody close to him, it is foolhardy to try to protect them from the truth. Just as you needed to know about your child's disability from doctors and nurses, your child, too, will need you to be honest with him and sensitive to his feelings. So tell him what you know, when you know it. Do not avoid telling or showing your child the reality, just because you think that he will not fully understand or that he may display unmanageable behaviour as a result. Anger is a typical reaction for some people and just because they have a learning disability does not mean that they should be rebuked or taken to task for responding in this way. On the contrary, just like anyone else, they need a degree of sympathy and understanding. Simply because they are unable to talk or express themselves well, or have profound intellectual disabilities, does not mean that they cannot feel grief. Whatever the extent of your son or daughter's disability, he or she will still need to go through the same mourning process as yourself, although he may very well show it in quite different ways.

Choose your words carefully

Using euphemisms like 'has gone to sleep' or 'passed over' serve only to confuse and delay full understanding of the situation. It is always better to use words like 'dead' and 'died', explaining exactly what they mean—that the dead person cannot come back or be with them any more. Remind them of those things which you should have been teaching them from a young age—that death happens to us all and that it is something of which we need not be frightened. All children need to become acquainted with death as it happens, so that early on they understand the whole cycle of birth, life and death. These are the basic facts of life and throughout their childhood, as they grow up, you will need to prepare them for these realities that they will one day surely encounter, whether you want them to or not.

Since the process of dying is happening around them all the time anyway, it is useful to use some of these opportunities to point out the inevitable to them from time to time. It needs to be done in a matter-of-fact way, rather than frightening the life out of them or continuously harping on about it in some morbid fashion. The deaths of famous people covered in the media, for instance, can sometimes be used. Flowers that bloom and die, neighbours' pets that shuffle off their mortal coil and so on. I am by no means proposing that you constantly dwell upon the morbidity of dying, but simply suggesting that making death a taboo subject for your child is going to stack up a few emotional problems for him or her at some stage in the future.

We need to understand, too, that both children and adults grieve over the loss of objects as well as people and animals. Often this can be felt just as intently as the loss of someone in their lives, sometimes even more intently. If you have ever lost or mislaid your purse or wallet, you will have some idea of the panic and anxiety that it can cause. Losing a favourite toy may seem trivial to an adult, but quite devastating to a child.

People who have learning disabilities may need to be told several times and in different ways before they completely understand the situation. Tell them even if they cannot use words themselves or seem as if they will never understand. If your son is able to speak or express himself in some way, he will certainly need opportunities for doing so. Many people who have learning disabilities find it hard to get their friends and family to listen to them properly. This is extremely frustrating for them at the best of times, but when they are in mourning it becomes unbearable.

Let them experience the practicalities of dealing with death

Do not try to find somewhere else for your son or daughter to be placed in order to leave you the space to get on with preparing funeral arrangements. Try to keep your youngster around with you, even if it means finding another person to help you cope. Registering deaths, clearing houses, destroying old clothes and so on are some of the practical processes which enable you to go through part of your own grieving and acceptance. Your child needs it too. He or she will also need to experience this atmosphere, in which people are generally sadder and more subdued in their manner than usual. It is all part of beginning to understand the reality of what has happened.

It is often even more important for people who have learning disabilities to have the opportunity to attend the funeral and perhaps spend time saying their goodbyes to the body of the deceased, especially if it is someone who has been very close to them. Make certain, too, that they get a chance to do things like buying their own wreath, rather than having their name attached to flowers from someone else, without even knowing it. These gestures help to make them fully aware of the reality of their loss. Of course, you and others who were close to the deceased person will want to take part in the funeral service without having to worry unduly about the day-to-day needs that have to be taken into account for someone who has learning disabilities—things like easy access if he or she has mobility problems, and so on. It is therefore a good idea to ask a reliable friend to take responsibility on the day, to ensure that the person with disabilities has all his or her basic requirements taken care of as and when necessary.

Never assume that you know how they are feeling

It is unwise to make assumptions about your son's or daughter's feelings, based upon the way that you yourself feel. Not only is everyone different in this respect, but the degree to which loss is felt depends upon your own particular relationship with the deceased, the regularity with which you used to see them and the degree of bonding that has taken place between you. You will feel the loss of a wife or a husband quite differently from the way your son or daughter will feel the loss of a father or mother. No matter what degree of intellectual ability a person may have, nobody can predict how he or she will react to a loss. For a child, losing a pet rabbit can be far more traumatising than losing an aunt or uncle. Feelings of grief can be incurred when members of staff leave a school or neighbours move away from your area, and it is often helpful if they can be encouraged to write a letter or perhaps make the odd telephone call from time to time, for a few months following their absence.

It is completely wrong for us to assume that a person cannot feel grief simply because he is unable to express his feelings of loss. All of us have feelings, irrespective of our abilities, and these include feelings of desperate sadness as well as great happiness.

Of course, not everybody will grieve about the same things. You may feel that they should or shouldn't be grieving about a certain person or circumstance, but your judgements about what they ought to feel will often bear little relationship to what they actually feel. If they are not grieving, then why make them grieve? If they are, then it is unwise to try to stop them. Attempting to jolly them up or get them to put a brave face on it will ultimately help no one.

Express your own feelings openly

Don't hide your feelings of grief from your children. Often we seem to think that there is something wrong about allowing ourselves to cry when they are around. It is better to share your grief with your children, rather than trying to hide it from them, which, in practice, you are rarely able to do very successfully anyway. It is better that children understand that other people feel the same way as they are feeling, rather than think that they are the only ones who are experiencing emotional pain—or even worse, learn that it is not good to express their sadness publicly.

Don't attempt to deceive

Never try to hoodwink a person by pretending that a loved one who has died is still alive or has gone away somewhere for a long time. Not only is there bound to be someone who lets it slip, but you will be depriving them of the whole grief process and will potentially cause them a considerable emotional upheaval which can become problematical and quite complex.

Keep giving your support after the funeral

Just as a physical wound takes time to heal, so it is with an emotional hurt—it may also leave a scar. A person's state of mourning doesn't end when the funeral is over, and he or she will need to have plenty of support from those round about in order to work through the various stages of grief mentioned earlier. Make certain that those who come into regular contact with your son or daughter know exactly what the situation is and advise them how they might deal with any difficult moments should they arise. If your child wants to, allow her to keep talking about the person who has died, and share memories of some of the times past, particularly the fun times. Look at old family videos together and talk over photographs. Some people shy away from doing this kind of thing with someone who has learning difficulties, in case the person becomes obsessive. This is nonsense; we are all much the same inside and need to feel that we are still somehow in touch with those who have gone, even if it is only being able to be in touch with the memories that they generated. My mother still talks to my father's photograph as if he is still there, and that's some seven or eight years now since he died. Nobody thinks this is in any way out of the ordinary. People with learning difficulties need to be able to do these sort of things, too, without their friends and relations reaching for the phone to call the nearest psychiatrist. Grieving for someone who has died is as much a normal part of our lives as is celebrating the birth of a baby. To preserve a balance in our own mental health, we need to have access to those emotional mechanisms within us, which allow our expression of sadness in the same way that we show our joy and gladness.

The process of grieving is likely to be a long one and can easily continue in some form for at least two or three years. Physically, intense emotion is extremely tiring, and allowances should be made for rest when it is needed. A person has not fully recovered from her trauma until she is able to live her life fully and independently of the one who has died. Living totally in the past, and continually organising all one's day-to-day events around considerations for the deceased, means that the griever is stifling her own existence. As the intensity of her loss subsides she must be encouraged to grasp the opportunities of developing some fresh interests and new relationships, which will help to make the rest of her life rich and meaningful.

When a death in the family occurs, as it surely will, all the other members of the family will themselves be grieving and in a state of mourning. Whilst family members will undoubtedly give and receive a good deal of emotional support among themselves, much of it will also need to come from friends. This is yet another reason why it is so necessary to have established a strong independent circle of friends for your son or daughter, as mentioned in the earlier chapters. There is no practical way in which we can fully prepare ourselves for the death of those who are close to us, even though it is so inevitable. However, a good social presence and a sound network of friends are essential if your son or daughter is to receive every help in overcoming his or her inner hurt. When your children come to mourn your own death, you need to be certain that someone will be there to offer them a shoulder to cry on. Nobody really wants to have to carry on alone.

12 Planning for When You'll no Longer be Around

> 'For the cause that lacks assistance, for the wrong that needs resistance,
> For the future in the distance, and for the good that I can do.'
>
> John Bampfylde

So many parents who have a son or daughter with learning disabilities say that their greatest wish is to outlive their children. This is a sad and sobering statement, and a very real indictment upon the services which are currently provided. It means that, through their direct experience of professionals and the support which they provide, many parents have learned to have precious little confidence in relying upon professional support to enable their son or daughter to live a happy and fulfilled life. This is so strongly felt by parents that they believe, quite vehemently, that their sons and daughters will be better off dead than having to rely entirely upon these services once their parents have gone.

But of course, most parents do die first and if they are to do it with some peace of mind they will need to give sufficient consideration, early on, to some of the key concerns about what will happen when they are no longer around. First, it should be understood that, no matter who we are, none of us should have to depend entirely upon our parents in order to live a full life. If we do, then effectively our meaningful life will come to an end at the same time as our parents' and that is both a nonsense and quite unacceptable. Becoming to some degree more self-determining in what we do and who we meet is essential if we are to live our lives in any meaningful sort of way. Some people will aspire to greater degrees of control over their own destiny than others, but if our goals really are to afford everyone the chance to have more choice, equal opportunity and to become as self-sufficient as possible, then the extent of their disabilities will, in effect, make no difference. We simply have to ask ourselves about each individual: what will it take, in terms of support, to enable this person to live his or her life to the full?

Judith Snow cannot move any part of her body other than her right thumb with which she has learned to manoeuvre her wheelchair. This does not prevent her from travelling regularly across the Atlantic to lecture on INCLUSION. Similarly, when Bernard Brett was alive, being unable to speak or move by himself led to him becoming institutionalised by the system for the early part of his life. However, his mother's commitment to teaching him how to communicate his thoughts and ideas by pointing his finger at letters of the alphabet which she printed on a card, finally enabled him not only to take charge of his own existence long after she died, but also meant that he could help others. After she died, Bernard lived in the house that his mother left him, and although he depended entirely upon others for all his bodily and functional needs, at the same time he managed to run a successful charitable organisation for people who were homeless. He became so proficient in spelling out his conversation on the card his mother had provided that, like many others, I often had to ask him to slow down, since he could spell out words faster than I could read them. Once I remember asking him why he didn't bring himself into the twentieth century by getting a computer, so that we could read more easily what he was saying on screen. Bernard pointed to the card on his lap and spelled out: 'Because then I would no longer have the advantage.'

If anyone lived a full life it was surely Bernard, who not only satisfied his own needs, but contributed a great deal to his local community by becoming an active member of the Community Health Council and various other local committees of that ilk. In his early forties he met and married an extremely attractive young woman, which was publicised in the local newspaper. I bumped into him in the high street shortly afterwards and said to him with a grin:

'I see that you have married a beautiful young woman almost half your age, Bernard. Do you know that this could be rather life-threatening?'

Bernard took hold of his card inscribed with the alphabet and proceeded to spell out, 'Well, if she dies, she dies.'

Whilst Bernard was always totally dependent upon others to cope with his physical day-to-day needs, he did not allow this to prevent him calling the shots when it came to making his own choices and decisions. His mother had managed to open up a channel of communication which nobody else had even suspected was possible, but more than that, she also encouraged him to take some control over his own destiny. She did not stifle his opportunities by interfering too much, although I'm sure that there must have been many times when she almost bit her tongue clean off in an attempt to prevent herself from interjecting and moulding Bernard's life in a way that she thought might be best. As a result, Bernard learned how to live his own life long before his mother died, which meant that she departed in the satisfied knowledge that her son was at least going to have the same chances in life as anyone else. One system which can lend itself to putting the person who has additional needs in the driving seat is Service Brokerage.

The benefits of a service brokerage system

These days, influenced by legislation from central government, Local Authorities and Health Services are undergoing a cultural change in their thinking about how they should plan and manage the services which they provide for us. They are being asked to do this in the same way that people in business run their companies. This does not mean that they should be measuring caring in terms of profit and loss, but rather that they should start to address themselves more fundamentally to analysing the way in which a healthy economy works and discover how this could be used to the best advantage for those who use their services. In the commercial field, business people know that they have to satisfy their customers if their company is to survive and go from strength to strength.

Take the motor industry, for instance. Last year it spent million after million on market research, in order to determine just what it is that its customers really want from their environmentally unfriendly mode of transport. Potential buyers were asked what shape car they liked best, what colours they preferred, whether they wanted performance or comfort from their car. The questions were both broad and specific. But, then, it is really only common sense to ask people what they want before you attempt to give it to them. After all, if they didn't like it, or if it didn't meet their needs, they wouldn't bother to buy it, and car firms would be left with a huge pile of unwanted rubber and metal on their hands.

So if we can do this for cars, why is it that we seem unable to do it for people? Why don't we ask them what they need *before* we give it to them, rather than telling them what we think they need and then giving it to them come what may? Now that the government has introduced this commercial culture into our human services, some administrators are beginning to examine the financial mechanics of what we often call 'the real world', and apply the advantages of it to people who have learning disabilities and their families, so that they can begin to gain some benefit. In the commercial world of high street shops, if we don't see what we want, or are not completely satisfied with what is being offered, then we don't buy, and if enough customers do this, eventually that business will go to the wall. In human services, however, it is quite different. There, we have no purchasing power whatsoever and have to accept everything that we are given or do without. Under these circumstances, it is the consumer who often goes to the wall, whilst bureaucracies, which provide, flourish.

The idea of Service Brokerage originated in Vancouver, Canada, in the 1970s, from parents of children with profound disabilities. The idea is to allow individuals to put together their own tailormade support system, which will give them the chance to live their lives in the way that they wish. To finance this properly, money is deflected from the usual investment into segregated buildings of one sort or another and from the high salaries that some administrators have been enjoying, and placed directly into the hands of those people who have additional needs, so that they can have what they want, when they want it.

Here in the UK people are beginning to recognise the enormous benefits of operating such a system. In an article written recently for *Community Living* magazine entitled 'Money For A Change?', David Brandon tells of a group of severely disabled people who were living in a nursing home run by a voluntary organisation. These people approached their District Social Services and asked them if they could be granted the same amount of funding which they were currently paying for the nursing home, so that it could be used to buy the lifestyle that each of them really wanted. This was agreed and, eventually, every one of them got the home and life of their own choice. The provider/purchaser framework under which Health and Social Services now operate lends itself particularly well to funding the needs of individuals in this way.

There are numbers of disabled people now who take direct responsibility for planning the purchasing of their own support needs. To do this, they often form themselves into a trust, in order to become eligible to receive grants. Well, if hospitals can become trusts, why not individuals? Such a trust can be made up of four or five people (or any number of people that you like) who take on the primary responsibility to see that the person in question has his or her wishes carried out and that the money allocated is spent according to these wishes. Thus accommodation, transport, and paid companions are employed on the person's behalf. Even though the individual may have considerable disabilities and be highly dependent upon members of his Trust to work on his behalf, the structure of this system leaves no doubt whatsoever about who it is all for and whose needs have to be met.

In parts of Canada a Service Broker exists, whose task is to lend assistance and advice independently, where it is required, to disabled people who seek help in buying in various supports which will enable them to achieve their desired outcomes. Whilst they are available if required, Service Brokers are not a compulsory feature of this system and will only lend a hand when, or if they are asked. Service Brokers are not part of the establishment and, as such, they are in a good position to help in the design of a personalised service which will meet the particular needs of the person for whom it is intended. Service Brokers have no part to play in making decisions; they merely help an individual to think his situation through and try to turn his wishes into reality.

This compares most favourably with our more traditional forms of support in which, all too often, professionals of one sort or another seem to end up taking over all the important decision-making and giving people very little of what they actually want or need. Unlike traditional formats, the Service Brokerage approach affords individuals respect and status, gives them the opportunity to fulfil their dreams and empowers them to become self-determining in planning and indulging in the lifestyle of their choice.

THE ADVANTAGES FOR INDIVIDUALS WHO HAVE LEARNING DISABILITIES

- People have direct control over their own lives.
  Disabled people will not find themselves forced into a role subservient to professionals.

- They have instant access to whatever support they decide they need.
  They will no longer have to be at the mercy of long waiting lists, appointments and so on.

- People have a much greater choice.
  It is a system which is truly needs-led as opposed to resource-based.

- The status and prestige of individuals is raised.
  It is the person who is disabled who calls the shots, since he or she holds the budget.

- The system has an in-built quality assurance.
  What people don't want, they won't have.

- Encourages those who provide services to be more efficient and to address needs better.
  Services which are not needed, too expensive or of poor quality, will not be purchased.

- It is flexible and easily adaptable.
  Support can be changed as and when an individual's needs change.

THE ADVANTAGES FOR LOCAL AUTHORITIES

- It is truly in keeping with their Care in the Community philosophy.
  Individuals become masters of their own destiny and have the resources to participate in the everyday routines, events and activities within their local neighbourhood.

- They will be certain that the needs of the individual will be properly met.
  People know best about their own needs and this system directly provides them with the resources to ensure that they can get access to exactly what they want.

- They will have a fixed expenditure without the liability of overheads.

This system operates like a cash grant, which means that there are no hidden costs for the Local Authority.

- They can get access to statistical information in respect of service-users' preferences.
  It is a simple process to do some market research on how people spend their grant allocation, which will in turn make Local Authorities aware of the trend in people's needs. This can have implications on future training courses and so on.

- No building maintenance costs.
  Since all monies under this system are paid in the form of individual grants, there is no money unnecessarily wasted on building programmes.

- No staffing outlay or personnel liabilities.
  Since all monies under this system are paid in the form of individual grants, the personnel liabilities become a matter for the individual or his or her trust.

- No legal liability for the services which are provided.
  Unlike the traditional system, where Local Authorities are always potentially liable.

- It encourages the creation of a whole range of alternative provision.
  Current provision is notoriously narrow, but under Service Brokerage, in which finance is dispersed to a number of individuals, the diversity of their needs means that a diversity of alternative provision will develop from a whole range of new enterprises.

- It is a system which can be extended to anyone who has additional needs.
  Service Brokerage can be applied to anyone who has additional needs—people who are elderly, people who have a mental illness and so on.

Under the Service Brokerage system, there is nothing to prevent individuals from pooling their funds in order to share costs and get more for their money. The flexibility of the system, combined with the fact that people have the option to take complete control of their own affairs, makes Service Brokerage an attractive proposition. Already more than 300 people in the United Kingdom now have direct control over their own support systems, using money allocated to them by their Local Authority. It is true that most of these people have physical disabilities and have chosen to opt out of the traditional services that they once received. However, there is nothing to stop this happening for those who have learning disabilities, particularly since a good many Social Service Departments seem to regard the Service Brokerage system as cost-effective and generally beneficial for all concerned. If you are interested in developing this idea further for your son or daughter, it would be advisable for you to join forces with others of the same mind and make an approach to your Local Authority with a view to developing a pilot study, using just a few people. Some pilot studies have already taken place in the UK, and currently Althea Brandon is in the process of setting one up in the Cambridge area (see address list at the end of this book).

Good parents do their level best to prepare their children for adulthood, when they will have to cope independently with all that the real world outside throws at them. If your son or daughter has additional needs, one of the greatest gifts you can make is to assist him in establishing himself in a system like Service Brokerage, where he can have a greater chance of living the life he chooses, with meaning and fulfilment. By the same token, as a parent approaching elderly status, you will be happier in the knowledge that your son or daughter has an effective and practical model of support which operates well for him or her. Seeing it function well and effectively whilst you're alive is the only way that you can have real peace of mind.

Brothers and sisters

In effect, whether they like it or not, or even realise it or not, when parents die they not only leave behind their disabled son or daughter, but they also pass on ownership of responsibility for them to any surviving brothers and sisters whom he or she may have. Some parents express their pride that a brother or sister, even during early childhood, demonstrates a strong willingness to care for a disabled sibling. They feel a little more reassured about the future when they hear their other child say, 'Don't worry Mummy, I'll always see that she comes to no harm.' By the same token, other parents do their best to prevent their other children from developing a feeling that they must always be responsible for their brother or sister's welfare.

Either way, it seems to make very little difference in the long run. Those who have a brother or sister who has additional needs are likely to feel much the same blood ties as their parents, no matter what you do. When parents give birth to a child who has additional needs, they know full well that this child is part of them and of their flesh and blood and, because of this, most people have a feeling, deep down inside, that they have no emotional alternative but to care for their child and to commit themselves to looking after his or her best interests for the rest of their lives.

It is a commitment that most people cannot help but make, even if, at the same time, they are resentful that it should have happened to them and really don't know how, or if, they are going to cope. They often feel tremendous undercurrents of anger, knowing that their life is going to change radically, but at the same time feel guilty for feeling this way—after all, it is hardly their child's fault. Then, since families seem to get very little practical help, some of them decide, through pure emotional and physical exhaustion, that they have no option but to consider handing their son or daughter over to some form of residential care. Coming to terms with doing this (if indeed anyone ever does) is agonising and emotionally very damaging.

Just as children with disabilities are born to parents, they are also born to brothers and sisters, which means that their brothers and sisters are likely to develop, as they grow up, the same internal struggles as their mother and father. If your disabled brother has always lived with you and your parents and your parents die leaving him alone in the house and unable to cope, then emotionally you are likely to find yourself pulled in different directions, in just the same way that your parents were. Even if you feel that you want to offer your brother or sister a place to live in your home, what will your wife or husband feel about it, since in practical terms she or he will have to share the coping? After all, unlike you, they have no blood ties.

The ramifications of passing on the responsibility of caring can be considerable. Therefore, as your disabled son or daughter grows up, the whole family needs to plan ways in which he or she can develop a system of support, which will not just provide independence and a lifestyle of his or her own, but will also give the brothers and sisters the opportunity to see that their sibling is safe, well settled and living a full life. Getting together a workable system which enables your disabled son or daughter to live independently of the family whilst you are alive, means that everyone in your family can live their own lives, satisfied in the knowledge that all is well and will continue to be well.

Making a will

Most of us simply don't like to dwell too long upon matters which remind us of our own inevitable demise, and for this reason we tend to put tasks like will-making to one side, even though we know that dying intestate could cause untold difficulties and inconvenience for those we leave behind. Some of us feel that we are too young to make a will and plan to consider such things later in life, when in fact we never really know just how much later we can afford to leave it. Others avoid the whole business altogether, by convincing themselves that they have nothing to leave anyway, although in fact most of us have something to bequeath.

Most people need to get their affairs in order, if for no better reason than to see that their life's savings aren't just reeled in by some government department. As the saying goes, we come into this world with nothing and we go out with nothing, so we ought to make the residue that we create between times available to someone who can use it well.

Having said that, I'm told (on dubious authority) that, a few years ago, a banker died, having previously given clear instructions to his solicitor that he wanted all his assets converted into sterling and placed in the coffin with him. Contrary to the old saying that you can't take it with you, this banker, it seemed, had planned to do exactly that. Nevertheless, even he was completely foiled by a quick-thinking relative who, just before the burial took place, wrote out a cheque and exchanged it for the cash. I cannot of course vouch for the accuracy of this story, but I do know that making a will is a common-sense thing to do; it is not expensive and can save those whom you leave behind a great deal of trouble.

When making your will, be sure to do it through a solicitor rather than trying to save money by writing it yourself. Too many people have not had their wishes met, simply because they thought that they would try to save a pound or two.

If you are planning to leave your assets to your son or daughter who has learning disabilities, then often the wise thing to do is to leave it in the form of a trust rather than directly to your son or daughter in person. In this way, the trustee or trustees become the legal owners of the bequeathed assets but can only use them to benefit the person for whom they act. You can design your trust in any number of ways to suit the needs of your own family's situation. For instance, some trusts allow the trustee to use both the capital and the revenue, whilst others decree that only revenue can be utilised. This means that the property itself can be maintained intact, so that it can be passed on to others, like brothers and sisters or their surviving children (known as residuary beneficiaries), at a later date, when the original beneficiary has himself died.

Choosing a group of trustees is of course pretty crucial. They not only have to be people whom you know can be trusted to carry out your wishes, but they also have to be younger than you, at the time of writing your will, in order for them to be likely to survive you. You can of course use a firm of solicitors or perhaps a solicitor in conjunction with a relative. However, you need to be aware that legal eagles rarely carry out their tasks and responsibilities for free. Your friendly bank manager will also be pleased to act as a trustee; however, banks' fees tend to be even higher than those of solicitors. Brothers and sisters of your disabled son or daughter can make excellent trustees, particularly when organised together with a firm of solicitors. Of course, you do not have to form a trust through a will: you can create a trust for your son or daughter at any time.

Bequeathing assets to your son or daughter who has learning disabilities can be a lot more difficult than you might think. If he is in receipt of income support, housing benefit or any other State benefits, he will lose them completely if, by leaving him money or property, you cause his savings to total £8,000 or more. He will also have his benefits reduced on a sliding scale if he has between £3,000 and £8,000. So anything left to your child over £3,000 may in fact become quite a disadvantage. Added to this, if he is living or is likely to live in accommodation provided by the Local Authority, either directly or through a private or voluntary organisation, then the Local Authority can deduct any amount that it sees fit from your son or daughter's personal wealth, in order to pay towards the cost of upkeep. Even if you leave assets only to your non-disabled sons and daughters, with an understanding that you expect them to make appropriate provision whenever necessary for their brother or sister,

Local Authorities can insist through the courts that money from your bequest is paid to them. Any money or assets that you leave in trust is also susceptible.

If you are the only surviving parent of a disabled person and fail to leave a will at the time of your death, this too can cause problems for your son or daughter. If you have a house or property or money which exceeds £3,000, the Court of Protection is likely to appoint a receiver on your son's or daughter's behalf, which will again undoubtedly lead to loss of benefits; and if your disabled son or daughter has to be placed in residential accommodation provided by the Local Authority, a charge will be made and taken from the bequest. The law, of course, is simply trying to ensure that those receiving benefits have no other assets to pay their way before the State forks out, but it makes no allowance for disability.

Therefore, under our present system, if you have a disability and very little income, you cannot receive large sums of money (unless they are very large) without eventually losing out and becoming poor again. Each family's situation is quite different, of course, but my own feelings are that it could be worth considering leaving your house (if you own one) in trust to your disabled son or daughter, with the idea of renting out some of the rooms to people who could be employed by the trust as live-in companions. These live-in companions would claim housing benefit to pay the rent which is paid to the trust and a small wage could then be paid to them from this amount. This means that your son or daughter could remain in your home (or another) after your death, being supported by a group of trustees who could employ live-in day-to-day help. These live-in companions would not be able to earn very much, but would have free accommodation as compensation. Where finances were tight, which tends to be the rule rather than the exception, trustees would do well to approach the local Social Services Department in order to negotiate a grant towards the cost of keeping your son or daughter in his or her own home. Social Services can sometimes prove helpful in this way, particularly when they realise that it is cheaper for them to offer a contribution towards costs, rather than be asked to take on total responsibility for the person themselves.

Making a draft life plan

Whatever your situation, it is always better to plan for your son's or daughter's future by considering things from his or her perspective. Start with your child, not with a building. Ask yourselves what it would take to enable your daughter to live in a home of her own and to do the things that she enjoys. Too many services for people who have learning disabilities begin by acquiring an empty property and then looking around to see who they can fit into it. Do not make the same mistake. It is the person who is important and the lifestyle that he or she wants, not the building. Ask yourselves, where is the best area for her to live? Does this area have all the facilities that interest her within easy reach, like a cinema, pubs and so on.? Do her friends live nearby? and so on.

Time passes quickly and children soon grow into adults. Most parents tackle their situation day by day, but it is important to address the needs of the future right now and have some vision of how it might look. If you want your son or daughter to have a lifestyle of her own, to have a degree of independence no matter how disabled she may be and if you want some peace of mind for yourself and a life of your own, then start straight away to draft out some general goals with the help of friends and family. Whilst your children are babies, map out a route that will enable them to have all the same experiences and opportunities as any other child. Resist placing them in a segregated special school and seek help from friends to work out ways of getting your child into his or her local mainstream school. Begin to drum up support from ordinary local people. Ask for their help and advice in overcoming difficulties that you face. These may be the people who will one day be trustees or advocates for your son or daughter.

As time goes on you will need to see that your child has chances to go to all the same places that other children of his or her age go to, make friends and acquaintances, send and receive invitations. Take reasonable risks and allow your child to learn from her mistakes, refrain from blaming all her behaviour on her learning difficulties, see her as a child first and disabled second and see that she has every opportunity to be included in all that is happening in her locality. With your friends and family, draft a rough life plan for your child and check it from time to time, so that you can see that you are on target for a good future. Your rough life plan may look something like this:

- Get a place in a local playgroup.
- Get a place in the local mainstream school with support.
- See that there is a chance regularly to have friends home in the evenings, weekends and holidays and for your child to visit friends regularly.
- Make sure that your child gets a place in the local secondary school with support.
- See that he or she has lots of opportunities to learn about a variety of interests and hobbies.
- Develop supported employment opportunities.
- Consider setting up a trust to develop a circle of friends, and to support your child in having a home of his or her own.

These are clear goals to keep you on target. You will not be able to attain them alone, but you will discover that ordinary people can accomplish extraordinary things if you only give them the chance by asking them to get involved and make the world a better place for your son or daughter.

Some Useful Addresses

The Centre for Studies on Integration in Education
415, Edgeware Road, London NW2 6NB.
Tel: 081–452 8642

PASSPORT Parents Group
1, Monfa Avenue, Woodsmoor, Stockport SK2 3SB.

Network 81
1–7, Woodfield Terrace, Chapel Hill, Stanstead, Essex CM24 8AJ.
Tel: 0279 647415. Fax: 0279 816438

Integration News
The Integration Alliance, 132, Wimbledon Park Road, London SW18 5UG.

Values Into Action
Oxford House, Derbyshire Street, London E2 6HG.
Tel: 071–729 5436. Fax: 071–729 0435

Status Employment
85, Waddon Way, Croydon, Surrey CR0 4HY.
Tel: 081–681 3178

The Centre for Integrated Education and Community—UK
7, Aspen Wood, Godley, Cheshire SK14 3SB.
Tel: 061–366 0200. Fax: 061–366 6460

The Centre for Integrated Education and Community—Canada
24, Thome Crescent, Toronto, Ontario, Canada.
Tel/Fax: 0101 416 658 5363

Community Living Magazine
Hexagon Publishing, 5, Dickerage Lane, New Malden, Surrey KT3 3RZ.
Tel: 081–336 0220

Learning Together Magazine
2, Devon Terrace, Ffynone Road, Ffynone, Swansea, South Wales SA1 6DG.
Tel: 0792 472562

Co-options Ltd
Morfa Clwyd Business Centre, Marsh Road, Rhyl, Clwyd, North Wales
Tel: 0745 330030. Fax: 0745 343135

National Development Team
Hester Adrian Research Centre, University of Manchester, Oxford Road, Manchester M13 9PL.

The Royal Association for Disability and Rehabilitation (RADAR)
12 City Forum, 250 City Road, London EC1V 8AF.
Tel: 071–250 3222

Opportunities for People with Disabilities
1, Bank Buildings, Princes Street, London EC2R 8EU.
Tel: 071–726 4961
Also at:
Birmingham: 021–331 4121. Bristol: 0272 856491. Manchester: 061–224 1743. Sheffield: 0742 723231. Gatwick: 0293 543388. Essex: 0277 201984.

National Children's Bureau
8, Wakley Street, Islington, London EC1V 7QE.
Tel: 071–278 9441

The Sports Council for England
16, Upper Woburn Place, London WC1H 0HA.
Tel: 071–388 1277

The Sports Council for Northern Ireland
House of Sport, Upper Malone Road, Belfast BT9 5LA.
Tel: 0232 1222

The Sports Council for Scotland
Caledonia House, South Gyle, Edinburgh EH12 2DQ.
Tel: 031–317 7200

The Sports Council for Wales
Sophia Gardens, Cardiff CF1 9SW.
Tel: 0222 397571

Independent Panel for Special Education Advice
12, Marsh Road, Tillingham, Essex CM0 7SZ.
Tel: 0621 779781. Fax: 0621 778070

SKILL National Bureau for Students with Disabilities
336, Brixton Road, London SW9 7AA
Tel: 081–274 0565. Fax: 081–274 7840.

Greater Manchester Coalition of Disabled People
11, Anson Road, Manchester M14 5BY.
Tel: 061–224 2722

Bibliography

The Turning Point, by Fritjof Capra. Fontana, 1983.

The Inclusion Papers: Strategies To Make Inclusion Work, by Jack Pearpoint, Marsha Forest and Judith Snow. Inclusion Press, 1992.

Everyone Belongs: Mainstream Education For Children With Severe Learning Difficulties, by Kenn Jupp. Souvenir Press, 1992.

Handle with Care, by Francis Owen. Gresham Books, 1984.

Action for Inclusion, by John O'Brien and Marsha Forest. Inclusion Press, 1989.

Putting People First, by David and Althea Branden. Good Impressions Ltd, 1988.

Living, Loving and Learning, by Leo Buscaglia. Souvenir Press, 1983.

Living in the Real World, edited by C. F. Goodey. Twenty One Press, 1991.

We Can Speak for Ourselves, by Paul Williams and Bonnie Shoultz. Souvenir Press, 1982.

Living Independently, by Ann Shearer. C.E.H. and King Edward's Hospital Fund, 1982.

What It's Like to be Me, edited by Helen Exley. Exley Publications Ltd, 1981.

Supporting Families with a Child with a Disability, by Alan Gartner, Dorothy Kerzner Lipsky and Ann P. Turnbull. Paul H. Brookes Publishing Co, 1991.

Support Networks for Inclusive Schooling, by William Steinbeck and Susan Steinbeck. Paul H. Brookes Publishing Co, 1990.

Coming to Terms with Mental Handicap, by Ann Worthington. Helena Press, 1982.

Parents and Mentally Handicapped Children, by Charles Hannam. Penguin Books in association with MIND, 1975 and 1980.

Disability Equality in the Classroom: A Human Rights Issue, by Richard Rieser and Micheline Mason. Inner London Education Authority, 1990.

Hope for the Families, by Robert Perske. Abingdon Press, 1973 and 1981.

Graphic Guide to Best Team Practices, by David Sibbet. Graphic Guides Inc, 1992.

Bringing Up a Mentally Handicapped Child, by Liz Thompson. Thorson's Publishing Group, 1986.

Seeking the Answers, by Kenn Jupp. Opened Eye Publications, 1991.

From Behind the Piano, by Jack Pearpoint. Inclusion Press, 1990.

Making the Right Start, by Sheila Jupp. Opened Eye Publications, 1992.

The Whole Community Catalogue, compiled and edited by David Wetherow. Gunnars & Campbell Publishers Inc, 1992.

Remembering the Soul of Our Work, edited by John O'Brien and Connie Lyle O'Brien. Options In Community Living, 1992.

New Life in the Neighbourhood, by Robert Perske. Abingdon Press, 1980.

Circles of Friends, by Robert Perske. Welch Publishing Co Inc, 1988.

Teaching Pupils with Severe Learning Difficulties, edited by Christina Tilstone. David Fulton Publishers, 1991.

New Directions in Education, edited by Ron Miller. Holistic Education Press, 1991.

Behind Special Education: A Critical Analysis of Professional Culture and School Organisation, by Thomas M. Skrtic. Love Publishing Company, 1991.

From Providing to Enabling, by Nirmala Rao. Joseph Rowntree Foundation, 1991.

Survey of Supported Employment in England, Scotland and Wales, by Tim Lister *et al*. National Development Team, 1992.

Am I Allowed to Cry: A study of bereavement amongst people who have learning difficulties, by Maureen Oswin. Souvenir Press, 1991.

After I'm Gone: What Will Happen to my Handicapped Child? by Gerald Sanctuary. Souvenir Press 2nd edition, revised, 1991.

Build Your Own Rainbow, by Barrie Hopson and Mike Scally. Mercury Books, 1991.

Direct Power—A Handbook on Service Brokerage, by David Brandon. Tao, 1991.

Building Community, by Ann Shearer. King's Fund Publishing, 1986.

PATH—A Work Book For Planning Positive Possible Futures, by Jack Pearpoint, John O'Brien and Marsha Forest. Inclusion Press, 1993.

Index